T0290640

China's Fight Against the COVID-19 Epidemic:

Its International Contribution and Significance in the Eyes of the World

Editor-in-Chief: Jiang Hui
Associate editors: Xin Xiangyang, Gong Yun
Edited by Li Ruiqin, Yu Haiqing, etc.

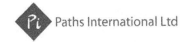 Paths International Ltd

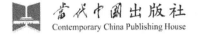 当代中国出版社
Contemporary China Publishing House

CONTENTS

Compiled Articles

FOREWORD

[China] Jiang Hui

July 2020, Beijing

Translated by Li Yi Finalized by He Jun

Tell the Stories of China's Fight Against the Epidemic and Strengthen Our Belief in the Four-sphere Confidence

Major risks and challenges in history invariably tested the comprehensive strengths of a country and nation and the governance capacity of its ruling party, and they also tested the strengths of the people as well as the state system. In 2020, an extraordinary year in the world history, the sudden outbreak of the COVID-19 pandemic has greatly impacted the work and life of humans, changed the economic and social trend, affected the development process of human beings, and is reshaping the political and economic order of the world. Amid this calamity, the concept of a global community of shared future has been severely tested and disseminated, and the strengths of the Chinese system have been fully manifested and won much recognition. It is an important task for theorists and cultural workers

1

in present-day China to artfully tell the world the stories of China's fight against the COVID-19 epidemic.

The CPC (Communist Party of China) Central Committee with Xi Jinping at its core has attached high importance to the crisis and major test caused by the COVID-19 epidemic. It has strengthened centralized, unified leadership over the prevention and control efforts, put people's lives and health first, and carried out the general principle of remaining confident, coming together in solidarity, adopting a science-based approach, and taking targeted measures. Thus a prevention, control and treatment system integrating central and local efforts under the unified central deployment was formed. The whole country was mobilized and the spread of the COVID-19 epidemic was quickly brought under control. The strategic achievements in China's battle against the epidemic added new chapters to the Chinese system, Chinese speed and Chinese spirit, fully embodying the maximum strengths of the leadership of the Communist Party of China (CPC) and China's socialist system.

Compared with other countries, China has demonstrated the following characteristics in its battle against the epidemic: First, adopt a commanding system integrating the central and local efforts and carrying out the work down to the grassroots level; second, maintain openness and transparency by timely making all kinds of prevention and control information known to the public, to interact with them and subject to their scrutiny; third, implement science-based prevention and control measures; fourth, grasp the key points while attaching equal importance to prevention and control, treatment and guaranteeing the supply of materials and funds; fifth, mobilize all people to jointly respond to the epidemic.

All these characteristics are concrete and vivid manifestations of the strengths of the socialist system with Chinese characteristics in epidemic prevention and control. Having withstood the test of the fight against the epidemic, the strengths of the CPC exercising overall leadership are further demonstrated, and so are the people-centered governance philosophy and China's ability to mobilize resources to accomplish major initiatives. Having passed the major test of the epidemic, the people have a better understanding of the leadership of the CPC and the strengths of the socialist system, and an enhanced sense of the Four-sphere Confidence, and have more faith in the bright prospect of the great rejuvenation of the Chinese nation.

The course of human development is always interwoven with the fights against global public health emergencies. As globalization keeps expanding in the world today, the outbreak of the COVID-19 pandemic poses an unprecedented huge challenge to global public health security. How to respond to a pandemic in the era of globalization? This constitutes a major test for international cooperation. Whether the COVID-19 pandemic can be more effectively brought under control worldwide depends on whether countries of different social systems and at different stages of development can come together to form a powerful synergy to jointly respond to the pandemic, in the process replacing disagreement with unity and prejudice with reason. As was pointed out by General Secretary Xi Jinping: "The human being belongs to a global community of shared future. Unity and cooperation are the most powerful weapon for beating an epidemic that has a direct bearing upon the safety of people in all countries." In the face of a raging pandemic, people share weal and woe. Only when all countries in the world voluntarily abandon disagreements between them, strengthen unity and cooperation, and join hands in their fight against the pandemic can they secure the final victory.

In the global prevention and control of the COVID-19 pandemic, the effective governance of China forms a stark contrast with the disorder of the West, and the development trend that the East rises while the West falls is further demonstrated. With the spread of the pandemic, chaotic situation appears as a result of ineffective governance in Western countries: infected cases keep increasing and hit record highs, the unemployment rates remain high, large-scale racial disturbances erupt frequently, and social rifts and unrests are increasingly aggravated.

Some Western politicians are scrambling to point fingers in an attempt to shirk their responsibilities for failing to bring the epidemic under control in their own countries, falsely accusing "China of being responsible for the epidemic," demanding that "China make an apology and compensate for their losses." They challenge the authenticity of China's data about fighting the epidemic, and claim that China is driven by "geopolitical motive" in rendering assistance to other countries and regions. A small number of Western parliament members and lawyers even file lawsuits against the Chinese government. These moves just wantonly vilify China, totally ignoring the fact that China has been effective in preventing the spread of the virus and bringing it under control.

Given the "noises" in the international society, China makes its stand clear: we firmly oppose any act of politicizing the epidemic or attaching labels to coronavirus; we oppose ideological bias, always unswervingly put into practice multilateralism, democratize international relationship, safeguard international fairness and justice, and unwaveringly follow the path of international cooperation for mutual benefit.

Since the outbreak of the COVID-19 epidemic, General Secretary Xi Jinping has attached high importance to domestic and international development of the epidemic, delivered important speeches on many occasions, and made important instructions. In his talks to leaders of foreign governments and international organizations, he emphasized that the epidemic knows no national borders or distinguish between races and is therefore the common enemy of mankind. He said that the international society should foster the awareness of building a global community of shared future, and "bolster confidence, support each other and join hands to make response, step up international cooperation in an all-round way, and rally strength to form a powerful synergy, so as to jointly win this battle against a major pandemic facing the mankind."

Following the guiding principles of the important instructions of General Secretary Xi Jinping and the unified plan of the CPC Central Committee, China constantly improves domestic epidemic prevention and control and treatment system. Based on that, it proactively promotes the international cooperation in epidemic prevention and control by sending medical teams to other countries and international organizations and provide them with funds and medical supplies, sharing experience on fighting the epidemic with the World Health Organization and the international community, and working hard to contribute its share to international joint efforts to combat the pandemic. Always upholding the vision of a global community of shared future, China and the international community support each other in their joint fight, fully presenting the image of China as a major country meeting its responsibilities.

As the most severe international public health emergency confronting human beings in 2020, the COVID-19 pandemic has become a focus of attention of academia abroad. Many of them have begun to ponder over some key theoretical and realistic problems. For instance, how to evaluate China's performance in its fight against the epidemic? How to explain the problems arising in the battles against the epidemic in some countries? How to weigh the impact of the pandemic on the global landscape and its future trend? How to understand the impact of the pandemic on the leftists in the world and the development of socialist movement? How to promote the cooperation in the global fight against the pandemic with the concept of a global community of shared future? They propound quite a number of targeted and foresighted views that are of international vision and profound in theoretical thinking.

To fully reflect these views, opinions and research findings, Research Center of Xi Jinping Thought on Socialism with Chinese Characteristics for a New Era, World Socialism Research Center, and Research Department of International Marxism of Academy of Marxism under the Chinese Academy of Social Sciences jointly study the subject by interviewing more than 20 foreign politicians and scholars and inviting them to make in-depth analysis and discussion on relevant issues and write 26 original articles from different perspectives. In addition, to give the readers a fuller picture of the latest studies by foreign scholars on the COVID-19 pandemic over the past six months, the research group has selected some important views from articles that have already been published, and summarized and commented on their views. Based on these efforts, the research group has compiled the book *China's Fight Against the COVID-19 Epidemic: Its International Contribution and Significance in the Eyes of the World.*

This book has the following characteristics:

First, the contributors are experts and scholars distributed extensively worldwide. Coming from 17 countries in Europe, Asia, North America and Latin America, including Italy, Spain, Germany, the US, Britain, Czech, Japan, Brazil, Austria, India and so forth, they are geographically representative.

Second, the interviewees in this book are mostly international leftist politicians and scholars who have lived for long periods of time in the capitalist world (The leftists from Eastern Europe have experiences of living under different social systems). Some of them visited China many times or once resided in China, others are experts who have long studied issues about China. In addition to professional academic background, they have profound knowledge about the situations in China and the countries where they live through comparisons and based on their personal experiences.

Third, these articles are problem-driven: the writers discuss and analyze major issues of universal concern amid our fight against the pandemic. In particular, proceeding from the comparison of the two social systems around the world and the perspectives such as building a global community of shared future, they put forward many objective, impartial, scientific, rigorous and thought-provoking opinions and views.

It is hoped these analyses and thoughts will help people have a better understanding of the fight against COVID-19 waged in China and the rest of the world, enable more people to learn about the true stories of the fight against the epidemic in China, and to be beneficial to further strengthening cooperation, expanding consensus, and making joint efforts to respond to the epidemic.

Feature Article

The World Landscape and the China-US Relations in the Wake of the COVID-19 Pandemic

[China] Li Shenming

Translated by Li Yi   Finalized by He Jun

About the Author

Li Shenming is a member of the Standing Committee of the 10th, 11th and 12th National People's Congress, deputy director of the Committee for Internal and Judicial Affairs of the 12th National People's Congress. He was a former vice president and deputy secretary of the Leading Party Members' Group of the Chinese Academy of Social Sciences, director of World Socialism Research Center, research fellow and tutor for doctoral candidates.

The sudden outbreak of the COVID-19 pandemic in 2020 has a huge impact on and long-term consequences for the world landscape, China-US relations and even global economy, politics, culture, trade, diplomacy, military affairs, education, and science and technology. Different attitudes demonstrated by different countries and political parties to the pandemic and corresponding measures they have taken give different revelations.

Correctly understanding the global landscape and managing China-US relations in the wake of the COVID-19 pandemic represent the overall planning for consolidating, improving, upholding and developing the top-level design of socialism with Chinese characteristics, represent how our comprehensive response will be under the changing domestic and international situation to ensure the fulfillment of the Second Centenary Goal – the Chinese Dream of the great rejuvenation of the Chinese nation, and it is also a glorious mission of the CPC in opening up new prospects in the history of human civilization and building a global community of shared future in a context of change at a level unseen in a century.

I. The world is entering a new age marked by major turbulence, major transformation and major development

Marx and Lenin compared social development to the obscured age when "twenty years equal one day" and the great days when "one day equals twenty years."[1] If the outbreak of the international financial crisis in 2008 unveiled a historical period marked by major turbulence, transformation and development, then the outbreak of the COVID-19 pandemic around the world in 2020 was an obvious signal marking the advent of this historical period. In a sense, the disaster is tearing the world apart, further intensifying the polarization between the rich and the poor, facilitating the awakening of people around the world and the progress of world history, speeding up the test of the respective strengths and weaknesses of socialist and capitalist systems, therefore accelerating the shattering of the illusion of some people that capitalism is the final destination of mankind. It is in this sense that we are entering a historical period undergoing change at a level unseen in a century, when one day equals 20 years.

In the world today, the objective conditions are available in many countries for the people to oppose oppression and exploitation, while the subjective conditions like theoretical preparations and the preparation of party organizations are far from being sufficient. The fight is not over yet. In his report to the 19th National Congress of the CPC, General Secretary Xi Jinping made a solemn commitment: "The

---

1   *Complete Works of Lenin*, Vol. XXVI, People's Publishing House, 1990, p. 78.

Communist Party of China strives for both the wellbeing of the Chinese people and human progress. To make new and greater contributions to humanity is our Party's abiding mission."[1] Only when the situations of the world, China and the CPC are placed in the context of this broad and severe historical background, can we better understand the lofty sentiment of General Secretary Xi Jinping when he made the powerful statement that "I will fully commit to the people and never fail them," and can we better recognize the weighty responsibilities undertaken by the Chinese communists and Chinese people.

II. The fight against COVID-19 is a full demonstration of China's soft and hard power, and China will surely hold dialogues with the US on a higher platform

In January 2020, the COVID-19 epidemic sounded again the alarm of the security crisis of the Chinese nation. Under the personal command and planning of General Secretary Xi Jinping and the firm leadership of the CPC, people of all ethnic groups across China are united, human, material and financial resources are mobilized, efforts are coordinated to wage a massive people's war in the new age, in which the strengths of the socialist system are brought into full play, and the pre-war mobilization mechanism and system in times of peace that have been formed over the past 70-plus years is continued and developed. We are convinced that the attempt of the American government of imposing maximum pressure upon us with the COVID-19 epidemic as an excuse will end up a complete failure, and we will be bound to secure a comprehensive and great victory against the COVID-19 epidemic in the end.

---

1   Xi Jinping, "Secure a Decisive Victory in Building a Moderately Prosperous Society in All Respects and Strive for the Great Success of Socialism with Chinese Characteristics for a New Era," *People's Daily*, October 28, 2017.

III. The outbreak and unchecked spread of COVID-19 pandemic across the world manifest the conflicts of financial imperialism at the deepest level

Classical Marxist writers did not discuss the relationship between capitalism and the plagues playing havoc with the human society. However, in his exposition on capitalism in 1867, Marx clearly pointed out: "The production of surplus value or making money is the underlying reason for this mode of production."[1] Engels pointed out in 1876: "When we investigate with careful deliberation nature or the human history or our own mental activities, what come into our sight first are pictures eternally interwoven by various links and interactions."[2]

For thousands upon thousands of years, viruses living as parasites to hosts have existed in nature. Why did one of them spread to humans in 2019 instead of any other year and runs rampant in the human society on a large scale in 2020? In the final analysis, producing surplus value or exploiting surplus labor are what capitalist production is all about, and are also the prominent manifestations of financial imperialism that represents the highest stage of capitalism. The number of viruses is increasing despite the progress in science and technology. People seem to be equal in front of viruses as viruses do not discriminate against one country or race in favor of another. However, people of different races in different countries live under different social systems and economic and social conditions, and they are therefore treated differently in the face of viruses. The responses made by various countries to the COVID-19 epidemic are completely different, reflecting in essence the differences in systems and values, and indicating the contrasts between priorities – prioritizing capital or prioritizing people's lives and health.

---

1   *Complete Works of Marx and Engels*, Vol. XLIV, People's Publishing House, 2001, p. 714.
2   *Selected Works of Marx and Engels*, Vol. III, People's Publishing House, 1995, p. 359.

IV. COVID-19 epidemic is bad, yet it can be turned into a good thing under certain conditions

Of course, the unexpected outbreak of COVID-19 is a bad thing for us. In a sense, the fight against COVID-19 represents a war in a broad sense. Without gunpowder smoke, the war has to be waged on an unprecedented scale. The initial passive response to COVID-19 soon turned into a battle of self-awareness. Such a change is an important indication that the Chinese people are clearly awakened. In his *On Protracted War*, Mao Zedong incisively pointed out: "Revolutionary war is an antitoxin which not only eliminates the enemy's poison but also purges us of our own filth."[1]

Taking advantage of China's hard struggle against the COVID-19 epidemic, the American government strikes blows to China, only to deliver a poor performance. After the COVID-19 epidemic runs rampant in the US, the responses made by the American government dumbfounded people all over the world, deeply revealing the decadent and declining nature of the capitalist system and values in the US, and further alerting and educating the ordinary people and officials in China. To uphold socialism with Chinese characteristics, we need negative examples like the Soviet Union where the Communist Party met its failure and the country was disintegrated. Likewise, we also need another negative example – the rude and unreasonable United States which preaches "democracy" and "freedom" day in, day out.

In a sense, if some Chinese are like the frogs boiled in "comfortable" lukewarm water, a large number of them would instinctively or be startled to jump out of the pot that begins to sizzle after the US delivered a blow to China when it was in difficulties. Some money worshippers who were hitherto only interested in climbing the career ladder and pursuing wealth for their small families are being educated on patriotism, collectivism, socialism and even communism. Having been tested and tempered by the COVID-19 epidemic, the whole Party will be bound to scale

---

1   *Selected Works of Mao Zedong*, Vol. II, People's Publishing House, 1991, p. 457.

new heights in terms of thinking, theories, organization, conduct, discipline and institutional development. The Party and the government will also be bound to reach a still higher level in terms of their governance capacity and the modernization of their governance system.

V. While socialism with Chinese characteristics marches on in triumph, the US is putting up a useless, last-ditch struggle

At the 43rd group study session of the Political Bureau of the 18th CPC Central Committee held on September 29, 2017, General Secretary Xi Jinping clearly pointed out: "Despite changing times and society, the basic tenets of Marxism remain true. Despite the tremendous differences between now and the days of Karl Marx, world socialism's 500 years of history shows that we are still where Marxism has said we should be." This is a very correct and important judgment deserving close attention and deep understanding on the part of the whole Party. At present, we are in an extended historical period of transition from capitalism to socialism, as was pointed out by Marx; at the same time we are in a shorter historical period of imperialism, as stated by Lenin; we are also in a still smaller historical period of transition from monopolistic, parasitic or decadent capitalism to dying capitalism.

It is obvious that the monopolistic international financial capitalism represented by the US is encountering an unprecedented major crisis unseen in a century, symbolizing the ultimate outbreak of capitalism's inherent basic conflicts between globalized production and private ownership of the means of production. Twelve years have passed since the international financial crisis broke out in 2008, yet the crisis is far from over, as a greater disaster is yet to come. While we are faced with many challenges, the US is encountering much tougher challenges that are fundamental in nature.

Some say the main reason for our success in bringing the epidemic under control is the strengths of our system and mechanism of mobilizing the manpower and resources of the whole nation and doing everything possible to accomplish a significant task. This answer is partly true. Our fundamental strengths lie in our people-centered philosophy, i.e., we do everything for the people and rely on them. The fundamental weakness of the West lies in that everything is centered on capital. In other words, in pursuing its own personal interests, the capital class depends on a tiny number of wealthy people who would scheme against each other when there is a conflict of interests among them.

Given the complicated international situation, the international struggles are entering an age of unrestricted warfare waged in all fields, directions and dimensions. On the one hand, we should dare to carry on struggles and secure victory; on the other, we should prepare ourselves for the darkness before dawn, prepare ourselves for responding to various kinds of desperate struggles to be waged inevitably by the imperialist America when it is dying, and prepare ourselves for cruel, bitter yet great and glorious struggles. The imposingly standing socialism with Chinese characteristics is the mainstay for ushering in the dawn of winning the progressive undertakings of mankind. In a sense, in the years to come when the US and China will be locked in a confrontation, it is China, in the final analysis, that is in control of this important period of strategic opportunity for development. The key lies in which country can outlast the other.

VI. As international situation begins to undergo significant changes, it is imperative to adjust China-US relations

The Trump administration published its first "National Security Strategy" on December 19, 2017, portraying China as a "strategic competitor" of the US. This is an inevitable outcome of the economic globalization and the deepening of the international financial crisis, the acceleration of the technological revolution led by the application of information technology and artificial intelligence, and the arrival of global multi-polarization and profound changes unseen in a century.

We should make corresponding responses when our opponent makes changes to their strategies and tactics. We will find a way out so long as we can make responses as required by the circumstances, otherwise we will fail in our cause. We should also attach importance to remaining unchanged on some matters amid the changes to be made. In a sense, it is the following things that will remain unchanged that determine the changes of the present-day world situation and the necessity of adjusting the China-US relations, and determine whether socialism with Chinese characteristics can stand firmly in the world now and in the future. The things that will remain unchanged mainly include the following 11 points:

1. The extended historical period of transition from capitalism to socialism as pointed out by Marx and the specific shorter historical period of imperialism as stated by Lenin remain unchanged.

2. The theoretical foundation laid by Mao Zedong for adapting Marxism to the Chinese context, the theoretical preparations he made for implementing the policy of reform and opening up, and the basic line of the primary stage of socialism as defined by Deng Xiaoping remain unchanged.

3. Taking a people-centered approach, which is the sole purpose and distinctive nature of the CPC, remains unchanged.

4. The fundamental principle that people and only people are the motive for creating world history remains unchanged.

5. The overall situation that world socialism is beginning to revive although it is still in low ebbs remains unchanged.

6. The fact that China is the largest developing country and the largest socialist country in the world remains unchanged.

7. The fact that the US is still the most developed capitalist country in the present-day world and that the American imperialism is in essence a real tiger and paper tiger at once remain unchanged.

8. The judgment that China is still in an important period of strategic opportunity when a great deal can be achieved remains unchanged.

9. China's sincerity and decisions of remaining committed to a basic state policy of opening up, promoting the development of an open world economy, coexisting peacefully with all countries in the world including the US and seeking cooperation for mutual benefit remain unchanged.

10. China's decisions that it will never seek hegemony, never engage in expansion, never give up its legitimate rights and interests, and never allow anyone to expect China to tolerate anything that undermines its own interests remain unchanged.

11. China's decisions of holding high the banner of peace, development, cooperation for mutual benefit, upholding justice on behalf of developing countries, and promoting the building of a global community of shared future remain unchanged.

The above 11 points have been directly or indirectly expounded or reiterated by General Secretary Xi Jinping following the 18th National Congress of the CPC. Reflecting the law of CPC governance, the law of building socialism and the law of the development of human society that have formed over a long historical period, these points echo each other, create a coherent whole, contain profound implications, and form organic systems with each other. They constitute an important component of the Xi Jinping Thought on Socialism with Chinese Characteristics for a New Era.

VII. We can place the hope of developing the China-US relations characterized by genuinely peaceful and friendly coexistence on the people of the US and China only

General Secretary Xi Jinping clearly pointed out: "People are the creators of history. They are the real heroes."[1] This is the core content of historical materialism.

---

[1] Xi Jinping, "Speech Delivered at the First Plenary Session of the 13th National People's Congress," *People's Daily*, May 16, 2020.

The Chinese history is created by the Chinese people; likewise, the world history is created by people across the world. The Trump administration represents the interests of a small fraction of monopoly capitalists. That's why the COVID-19 epidemic is spreading unchecked in the US. The chaotic measures adopted by the Trump administration in responding to the COVID-19 epidemic will inevitably intensify the basic contradictions between the socialized or even globalized production and private ownership of the means of production in the capitalist world, intensify the contradictions between the monopoly capitalists in the US and the American people or even the people in other countries, and intensify the contradictions within the Western world.

The global economy is expected to grow by -3.0 percent in 2020, and the forecasted growth may be reduced further. The month of March in 2020 witnessed four out of five circuit breakers occurring in the history of the American stock market. Even Warren Buffett, known as "the god of stock," said with mixed feelings that he had never seen anything like this over 89 years of his life. The settlement price of NYMEX WTI crude oil futures closed at -US$37.63 per barrel, with an intraday decline of more than 300 percent. George Floyd, a black American, died after he was pinned to the ground by a policeman with his knee. His death set off the largest protest against racial discrimination and the use of force in law enforcement over the past decades in the US, with impacts spreading across the world.

In *Manifesto of the Communist Party*, Karl Marx and Friedrich Engels clearly pointed out: " ... in times when the class struggle nears the decisive hour, the process of dissolution going on within the ruling class, in fact within the whole range of society, assumes such a violent, glaring character, that a small section of the ruling class cuts itself adrift, and joins the revolutionary class, the class that holds the future in its hands. Just as, therefore, at an earlier period, a section of the nobility went over to the bourgeoisie, so now a portion of the bourgeoisie goes over to the proletariat, and in particular, a portion of the bourgeois ideologists, who have raised themselves to the level of comprehending theoretically the historical movement as a whole."[1]

We are convinced that a number of progressive capitalist thinkers will align themselves with proletarians around the world as the international financial crisis further worsens in the next two or three decades or even half a century. We are further convinced that in the days to come, thanks to the strong and correct leadership of the CPC Central Committee with Xi Jinping at its core and the strengths of the socialist system with Chinese characteristics, the CPC members and the Chinese people will dare to and be good at waging a great struggle in the new historical stage, and they will surely be able to undertake the glorious and sacred mission of realizing the Chinese Dream of rejuvenating the Chinese nation, building a global community of shared future and promoting the progress of human civilization. Fundamentally speaking, only socialism can develop China and make it powerful, and only socialism can ultimately save and develop the world. The world around 2050 will surely usher in bright sunny days of socialism and a global community of shared future.

VIII. We must adhere to the principle of fighting and cooperating at the same time and seeking cooperation through fighting when developing the China-US relations

People often ask what we can do when the US clings to cold-war thinking although we strongly oppose it. No matter how things stand, suppose the China-US relations are defined as that of a "couple," then what we should do when we refuse to divorce although the US is determined to do so? For instance, it was up to the US to avoid conflict with China on the Korea Peninsula in the early 1950s. Will the China-US relations characterized by cooperation for mutual benefit be decoupled? We are unable to provide a definitive answer out of our good wishes

---

1   *Selected Works of Marx and Engels*, Vol. I, 1995, People's Publishing House, p. 282.

only. It is because of this that we should first and foremost dare to struggle, and we cannot assume that the US would cooperate with us for mutual benefit without our struggle. We must make every effort to secure our due rights while firmly refusing the unreasonable demands of the US.

Some people say we need to use our mind rather than flex our muscles and engage in a direct confrontation with American hegemony. In fact, when guarding our bottom line, we should not be intimidated by the Americans; we should dare to struggle even at the price of severing the relationship. This is where the greatest wisdom lies. Abandoning the bottom line that should have been guarded under the excuse of being wise indicates, to put it mildly, a state of muddle-headedness, and in essence, an act of treason.

Some others always mistake the aspect of "a real tiger" as the whole picture of the American hegemony, saying that "the present-day China can exert impact on the world, but it does not hold sway over it. At present the US is the only country that can hold sway over the world, and this is a fact we must accept." First, China always respects the wishes of people of all countries, believing that all countries, big or small, strong or weak, should coexist peacefully, that different civilizations should communicate with and learn from each other, and opposing any force that attempts to lord it over the world. Next, such a statement ignores the fact that the American hegemony is, in essence, "a paper tiger." This is tantamount to admitting that the US is allowed to lord it over the CPC, the socialist China and the Chinese people all at the same time. Such a statement is tantamount to admitting that we can do nothing but to surrender to the American hegemony. We can and will never accept such a logic.

To guard our strategic bottom line, we shall stand firm like a mountain despite winds and rains, and wage a tit-for-tat struggle to defend every inch of our territory. We are also aware that in addition to fighting fearlessly against American hegemony, we need to adopt a set of correct strategies and tactics. We should fight the US hegemony on just grounds, to our advantages and with restraint. Since our aim is to safeguard China's security and territorial integrity, we shall go all out to fight without taking unnecessary risks. We oppose both tactics of "cooperating in everything without putting up a fight" and "fighting on everything without cooperation."

The cooperation should be conducted in accordance with principles and in a proactive way, while concessions should be made with limitations and conditions. No compromise should be made in key places and fields. For instance, as finance is the bloodline of China's economy, we will never allow the US to insert too many blood-sucking tubes into the blood vessels of China. The blood-sucking tubes that have already been inserted should be resolutely pulled out wherever it is possible, and we should manage to control the switches of blood-sucking tubes where it is impossible to pull them out for the time being.

In the areas where concessions can be made, we should do it step by step after fighting instead of granting it to them on a plate. When making concessions in the field of trade, for instance, we can appropriately increase the amount of food, clothes and daily necessities we import from the US to ease the conflict between the two countries. However, we shall be prudent when it comes to the importation of genetically modified food, and shall refrain ourselves from depending on imported American grain. As the US still enjoys advantages in many fields of science and technology, we may appropriately increase our importation of hi-tech products from the US on the preconditions that the development and innovation in relevant hi-tech fields of China should not be obstructed and that the long-term reliance on American technologies should be avoided. We shall do our best to isolate diehards, win over the wavering middle-of-the-roaders, and rely on the progressive forces in the US, especially the American people. As the decline of the American hegemony is a relatively long process, seeking cooperation through fighting should be adhered to as a principle over the entire process.

According to some comrades, we can by no means merely rely on our hot-bloodedness when dealing with the US, and we cannot achieve glory unless we can endure the hardest of hardships. If we can keep a low profile for a few more years, we will gain further development and grow stronger to ensure the fulfillment of the Chinese Dream of great rejuvenation of the Chinese nation.

In my opinion, we should make a detailed analysis of the above argument rather than simply labeling it as soft or tough. We must maintain an unyielding stance on anything that touches our bottom line, while remain appropriately flexible on things where compromise is possible. We shall never give the American authority the impression that "fight, but do not break" is the bottom line of China and that the bottom line of China's national security can be traded, otherwise we will never be able to develop and grow in strength, but will end up going in the opposite direction of our good wishes.

General Secretary Xi Jinping emphasizes on many occasions that we should dare to fight. This statement also applies to and serves as a precondition for establishing sound and stable China-US relations. We shall not avoid the mention of fighting, because not being afraid to fight is always one of our fundamental strategic guidelines. We emphasize the necessity of daring to fight against the wrong thoughts within the CPC, let alone the fight against a small number of diehards in the US. There is every reason for us to dare to struggle, and we will make our bottom line known to people around the world clearly. Daring to struggle means that we shall not fear the decoupling of China-US relations, something a small number of American politicians have threatened to do. Under no circumstance shall we abandon the core interests in our territory and sovereignty; nor shall we abandon the core interests in opening up the financial sector, ideology and industrial innovation.

Of course, we always emphasize that daring to fight is not enough; we must be good at it as well. We shall wage struggles on just grounds, to our advantage and with restraint. Being skilled at fighting is actually an integral part of daring to fight. Only when we dare to fight can we hold fast to our bottom line, uphold the leadership of the CPC and the socialist system. Only when we dare to fight can we uphold justice on behalf of others, and unite most other countries and the majority of people in the world, including ordinary American people of all social strata except for an extremely small number of diehards in the US. Only when we dare to fight can we "drive a donkey to go uphill" (by Mao Zedong), and strive for the cooperation with the US for achieving mutual benefits. Only when we dare to fight can we win popular support in China and achieve the grand goal of building a global community of shared future by working together with people all over the world to overcome difficulties and obstacles. Otherwise we will end up with no support from the Chinese people and no friendship from people around the world.

Since the outbreak of the COVID-19 epidemic, the press spokespersons of the Ministry of Foreign Affairs of the People's Republic of China have refuted the lies of the American government and exposed its hegemonic nature. They have won positive responses from people in China and those concerned abroad. The groundless criticism of the Foreign Ministry spokespersons only serves to convince us about the importance and necessity of daring to fight and fighting through to the end. Therefore, we shall suspend the use of statements like "keeping a low profile" and "fight, but do not break." We shall never "keep a low profile" when it comes to our theories, guiding principles and strategies; instead, we shall make them known to all people around the world. On the other hand, we shall leave room for flexibility and mobility in the tactics we adopt. We shall never give the US the wrong impression that our bottom line can be bargained, and that "fight, but do not break" is our bottom line. We can reiterate, at appropriate times, that the bottom lines we have defined should not be overstepped, just as the 17th parallel north was defined by Mao Zedong as the line that should not be overstepped during the War to Resist US Aggression and Aid Vietnam.

IX. Hold high the great banner of a global community of shared future and forge a most extensive international united front against hegemony

The thought of General Secretary Xi Jinping on building a global community of shared future timely answers the call of the times, and occupies the commanding height of human civilizations and morality. It represents the achievements of human thinking and civilization as well as the weighty theoretical outcome of building and improving the most extensive international united front against hegemony. In essence, however, it inherits and develops the "real community" and "association of free individuals" as expounded in Marxism, or the communist thought that represents the maximum program and ultimate goal of communists.

At present, the foundation of the American hegemony is weak. Considering only the interests of a tiny group of international monopolistic capitalists, it is in essence going against the fundamental interests of the vast majority of people in the world. As a result, rifts begin appearing not only within the group itself, but also among its allies. With the decline of its influences, the US has already felt and will inevitably continue to feel anxious. By taking advantage of its hegemonic position in trade, military affairs, finance and intellectual property rights, the US demands its partners and allies to "unite" under its control, kowtow to it and pay tributes to it. As it creates turbulence and tension everywhere by wielding its stick, it is only encountering strong dissatisfaction from more and more countries and their people wherever it goes, which lays the fundamental political foundation that an international united front against hegemony can be established and consolidated.

An international united front against hegemony should be guided by a major country daring to uphold justice. In the late 1980s and the early 1990s, Eastern Europe underwent drastic changes, and the Soviet Union disintegrated. In view of the international situation at that time, it was quite right for Deng Xiaoping to timely put forward the strategy and guidelines of "keeping a low profile" and "never taking a lead." However, great changes have taken place in the international situation. The US regards China as its major opponent, and the countries in the Third World or even the Second World and their people are eagerly looking to the Chinese government to uphold justice for them in international affairs. At a prize-awarding ceremony held in the US on January 21, 2020, German Chancellor Angela Merkel appealed to major Western countries "to treat Beijing on an equal footing instead of shutting it out."[1] On January 18, 2020, Aung San Suu Kyi, state councilor of Myanmar, said to President Xi Jinping during his visit: "We hope China can continue to uphold justice on behalf of small and medium-sized countries like Myanmar in the international arena."[2]

The right *qi* exists inside; evils cannot make disturbance. A person's dignity should be defended first by the person himself. Daring to defend one's own dignity and bottom line instead of making unnecessary compromise sets an example for other countries in opposing hegemony. In addition, maintaining justice requires mutual support. Only when we dare to speak up for and give support to countries which are subject to bullying and intimidation and which find themselves in difficulties or crises, will these countries in turn speak up for us and give support to us when we run into difficulties. If we can closely rely on the large number of the countries in the Third World and the countries in the Second World by making full use of the broad stage of the United Nations to firmly give at least moral support to these countries and their people in their just struggles from every aspect and as much as possible, we can forge a most extensive united front against the American hegemony in the world.

At present, some individual country seeking hegemony is withdrawing from various international conventions that it deems unfavorable to it, or even from some agencies of the United Nations. We can bide our time or create conditions so that we make advances while the hegemony retreats. We should strive to promote the concept of a global community of shared future and relevant views of China around the world through the platform of the United Nations.

1　"Merkel: The West Should Treat China on an Equal Footing Instead of Shutting It Out," January 23, 2020, see: http://www.cankaoxiaoxi.com/china/20200123/2400789.shtml.
2　"Xi Jinping: China Will Continue to Speak Out in Defense of Justice for Myanmar in the International Society," January 18, 2020, see: http://news.sina.com.cn/c/xl/2020-01-18/doc-iihnzhha3295385.shtml.

Exclusive Interviews

The World Is Focusing on China

[Germany] Egon Krenz

Edited by Li Ruiqin[1] Wang Jianzheng[2]   Translated by Li Yi   Finalized by He Jun

About the Author

Egon Krenz was born in Kolberg (the region of Pommern within the territory of today's Poland) in 1937. Krenz served as the first secretary of the Central Council of the Free German Youth in the German Democratic Republic in 1983. From 1983 to 1989, he was a member of the Political Bureau and member of the Central Secretariat of the Socialist Unity Party of Germany. On the eve of the drastic changes in Eastern Europe in October 1989, he succeeded Erich Honecker as the general secretary of the Central Committee of the Socialist Unity Party of Germany, chairman of the Council of the State and chairman of the National Defense Council of the German Democratic Republic. After the fall of the Berlin Wall in November 1989, he resigned from all posts in early December 1989. After the German reunification on October 3, 1990, Krenz was tried and given a six-and-a-half-year sentence after being found "guilty" in 1997. He was released from prison in 2003.

1   Li Ruiqin, research fellow of the Academy of Marxism, Chinese Academy of Social Sciences.
2   Wang Jianzheng, senior advisor to China Institute for International Strategic Studies.

Abstract

The fight against COVID-19 in China fully showcases the institutional strengths of socialism. In contrast, seriously affected by ideological prejudices, the West fails to objectively assess the great efforts and achievements of China in its battle against the epidemic; and such failure indicates that the forces represented by the US are seeing their influences weakened worldwide and their global reputation decreased. The outbreak of COVID-19 worldwide alerts people again that the construction of "a global community of shared future" as advocated by President Xi Jinping has never been so realistic and urgent.

On April 4, 2020, the national leaders of China and people all over the country stood in silent tribute to mourn those who had given their lives in the fight against COVID-19, and those who had died of the disease, while air raid sirens and horns of automobiles, trains and ships were sounded. All public buildings across the country and Chinese embassies in foreign countries flew national flags at half-mast to mourn the dead. The entire world recognized that China is united even at its most difficult period of time, and the ordinary people, members of the Communist Party of China, and senior state leaders all stick together. Instead of the "nervous temperament" commonly seen in a capitalist country, what are demonstrated in China are optimism and courage, and what is communicated is the hope of being able to beat the virus.

I. China's battle against COVID-19 fully demonstrates the institutional strengths of socialism and the humanitarian principle based on socialism with Chinese characteristics

China contained the spread of coronavirus in less than two months, winning precious time for other countries including Germany to fend off the virus. China's efforts would be acknowledged by anybody without ulterior motives. The approaches and methods that China has adopted in its response to this global crisis demonstrate the institutional strengths of socialism. The old medical prescriptions made by the capitalist world are no longer welcomed, as the focus of the world is shifting. What lies at the core is the people-centered approach, not the profits of capital.

Only 80 million people would be involved if measures against COVID-19 are adopted in Germany, while in the US, the number amounts to 300 million. This number would rise to 1.4 billion in China, or 22 percent of the world population. This figure alone is sufficient to show how heavy the responsibilities that China is shouldering. China undertakes such responsibilities for the sake of the world at large rather than for its own sake only. The crisis poses a challenge to the entire world. Even the anti-China forces in the West which deliberately ignore this point cannot obstruct socialist China to play an important role in courageously taking its responsibilities and going all out to fight COVID-19.

Staying united with one heart is the paramount principle in the long-term strategy of the CPC. At the 19th National Congress of the CPC, General Secretary Xi Jinping depicted the long-range prospects for China in 2049, when the republic celebrates its 100th anniversary. He also pointed out all kinds of risks that may arise on the path of development. According to him, the world is faced with many instabilities and uncertainties, such as ecological disaster, global economic crisis, armed conflicts and major communicable diseases. These risks are beyond prediction.[1] Even all measures are taken to mitigate or eliminate these risks, there still exist the possibilities that unexpected emergencies may arise.

It was therefore stated in the report delivered at the 19th National Congress of the CPC that "We will promote safe development, and raise public awareness that life matters most and that safety comes first; we will improve the public safety system and the responsibility system for workplace safety; we will take

---

1   Xi Jinping: *The Governance of China*, Vol. III, Foreign Languages Press, 2020, p. 46.

resolute measures to prevent serious and major accidents, and build up our capacity for disaster prevention, mitigation and relief,"[1] so as to overcome all difficulties and obstacles that we meet on our way. Practices have proved that China has successfully contained the spread of COVID-19 by giving full play to the institutional strengths of socialism.

China's approach in responding to the crisis of COVID-19 stems from the humanitarian principle based on the socialism with Chinese characteristics. Any European citizens without prejudices would hold China in esteem, because China was able to build from scratch two emergency field hospitals for fighting against the epidemic within the minimum period of time. Such a life-saving struggle is consistent with the historical achievements of the CPC. It is with such a spirit that China has made it possible to lift more than 800 million people out of poverty over the past decades. What severe consequences that the communicable disease would have caused but for the life-saving efforts based on the trans-century social achievements obtained!

As is stipulated in the Constitution of the People's Republic of China, the socialist ownership of the means of production takes the forms of state-owned properties and properties collectively owned by the working people, which lay a foundation for maintaining China's economic order. All the natural resources, among other things, the land, waters, forests, mountains, as well as the goods, materials and services provided by the state, are owned by the state. All these are the prerequisites on which the subsistence of people is dependent. In the meantime, the national facilities for preventing and treating diseases are not in the possession of those seeking profits only. The capitalist world is no match for China, which enjoys this inestimable advantage. In my eyes, the key element lies in ensuring the provision for subsistence in the interests of people.

---

1   Xi Jinping: *The Governance of China*, Vol. III, Foreign Languages Press, 2020, p. 38.

II. The forces represented by the US are losing their influences worldwide

A man with ideological prejudices and an air of self-important arrogance, American President Donald Trump went so far as to label COVID-19 as "Chinese virus." He is most skillful at throwing blames to others. To cover up his own failure, he even criticized the World Health Organization (WHO) for understating the risks of COVID-19 out of its Pro-China position. At the time when the world was in urgent need of international cooperation, the US froze the funding for paying its outstanding membership dues to the WHO. Trump maliciously turned the mistakes of the US in fighting against the epidemic into an uproar for inciting nationalist sentiments and the activities promoting armament in NATO. This aggravates conflicts in a world that is already disintegrating. The forces represented by Trump are losing their influences and reputation worldwide. As a result, the risk that a new war breaks out is increasing. The military expenditures of the US run as high as US$700 billion, exceeding the total sum of the other 15 countries which are next only to the US in terms of military expenditures. In the crisis caused by the COVID-19 epidemic, the German government decided to purchase 45 American fighter planes that can carry nuclear bombs, and confirmed the perpetual rights of the US to deploy nuclear weapons on the territory of Germany.

In fact, the appalling slanders committed by Trump represent an attempt to cover up the social criminal behaviors in the US. The truth behind them is that the hard-pressed American medical system hinders those in need of rescue from finding effective channels of medical treatment. This indicates a state of social collapse, an unavoidable misfortune that will befall most people when they suffer from diseases.

Miseries were reported all over the world. For instance, in Bergamo, a city in Italy, convoys of military vehicles carried the corpses of the dead to crematories. Frozen corpses were stored in an ice sports stadium in Madrid, Spain. At the corridors overcrowded with patients at hospitals in Detroit, some patients were stifled to death, yet nobody there was allowed to calculate the number of infected cases or deaths. In contrast, China did everything it could to rescue those in need, in stark contrast to what was happening across the ocean.

III. The ideological prejudices of the West seriously prevent it from recognizing China's efforts and effectiveness in fighting the epidemic

While the European Union (EU) leaders were frantically quarreling among themselves as to what they should do to respond to COVID-19, some Western politicians claimed that China's aid to other countries in their fight against COVID-19 is but a publicity show. This ridiculous statement was made at a moment when honest people around the world shared the joy with the citizens of Wuhan when the city gradually returned to normal after a two-month-long lockdown. Then let's look at the facts behind the so-called "publicity show":

Even at a pivotal moment in its own fight against the epidemic, China actively gave assistance to other countries, going all out to help them stem the spread of the coronavirus. The doctors from China supported their colleagues in Russia, Cuba and Venezuela, and rendered aid to Italy, an EU country suffering from misery. In Munich, the governor of the State of Bavaria personally went to the airport to receive the medical equipment from Shanghai that was urgently needed in Germany. China provided timely help to Kreis Heinsberg, a county in North Rhine-Westphalia which was severely affected by coronavirus. In a public letter, the governor of Kreis Heinsberg sincerely expressed his gratitude to China for its medical supplies and his admiration about China's effectiveness in its fight against the epidemic. In his letter to Angela Merkel, Chancellor of Germany, President Xi Jinping said that China would provide assistance to the best of its ability to Germany. In sharp contrast, the EU presents scenes of misery: all countries close their land borders according to their own needs, compete against each other in purchasing face masks and protective clothing, and refugees are left at the mercy of fate.

As China poses a great challenge to the West in terms of its national strength, the anti-China propaganda organized by the West is intended to throw the blame of the outbreak of COVID-19 to China to contain China's development. While coveting the huge market in China, they are more fearful that China will become a realistic choice to replace the capitalist system that is already out of control.

Unfortunately, under the cover of "media freedom," German journalists joined an anti-China chorus demonizing China. The media war directed against China has gone beyond the limits of inciting racial hatred. Upon seeing the uproar, I recall the words of August Bebel (1840-1913), a revolutionary and cofounder of the Social Democratic Party, which mean that when you are praised by your enemy, it shows you must have done something silly. Today, a backward reasoning means that the more vicious and silly the attack launched by "neoliberalists" and their media against the Chinese policies, the more it proves that China is taking the right path.

IV. Constructing a global community of shared future has never been more realistic

Paul Robert Vogt, a cardiac surgery professor from Switzerland who maintains the closest academic contact with his colleagues in Wuhan, recently reproached "the stupid attack against China," and recollected the advantages of the favorable experience provided by China: "When China reported the information about the appearance of a new virus to the WHO on December 31, 2019, other countries had two months to study the accurate data and come to the right conclusion." However, the US ignored this period of time, and is attempting to shift the blames onto China.

In its extreme form, the coronavirus has taught humans a lesson: their ruling over nature has limitations. Just as what humans did in the past when they were confronted with crises, they must respond to the current crisis with an approach characterized by humanitarian principle and social responsibility. This is completely different from the smoke screen put up by the capitalism. The construction of a global community of shared future has never been more realistic. In such a spirit, the West should have lifted the sanctions against Cuba, Venezuela, the Russian Federation and other countries. Such sanctions have hindered the delivery of medical supplies and other aid goods and materials as well as the exchanges of professionals. This is a sheer absurd act without the least reason. China is highly acclaimed by the international society for voicing its view in the United Nations against the continuation of such sanctions.

When the COVID-19 pandemic is brought under control, the entire world will be faced with a number of problems: What kind of life do we hope to live? How to replace a world in which each tries to cheat the other with a world featuring unity and mutual help? The issue about social systems has been put on the agenda of the world. This is an important issue that all people should ponder over when China has emerged from the dilemma and made its choice. The socialism with Chinese characteristics has won reputation worldwide. China is marching on the path of socialism, and other countries will follow its steps.

A Pandemic Revealing Problems with the System*

[Germany] Hans Modrow

Edited by Li Ruiqin[1] Wang Jianzheng[2]   Translated by Li Yi   Finalized by He Jun

---

About the Author

Hans Modrow was born on January 27, 1928 in Jasenitz, Pomerania, Germany (now Western Pomerania, Poland). From 1971 to 1973, Modrow was the head of the SED's (Socialist Unity Party of Germany) department of agitation and, then until 1989, SED's first secretary in Dresden. From November 13, 1989 to March 18, 1990, Modrow served as premier of the German Democratic Republic (GDR) for four months. On October 3, 1990, the

---

*   This article was first carried on *New Germany* (*Neues Deutschland*) on May 12, 2020 under the title of "Nonsense! Chinese Pestilence – How COVID-19 Pandemic Highlights the Problems with the System." It was noted that the article was written at the request of the Chinese Academy of Social Sciences. The Academy hoped that celebrities of various countries could share their views and positions on the COVID-19 pandemic and the battle against it, and would publish a book that collects all these articles. On May 14, 2020, under the title of "Article by Modrow – Former Prime Minister of the German Democratic Republic – The Battle Against the Pandemic Highlights the Strengths of the Chinese System," an abridged translation of the article was carried on *Reference News* in China. It is praiseworthy for Modrow to courageously sing praise of China in the German media, to lead the Left Party to seek new directions of endeavor by seizing opportunities provided by the battle against the pandemic, and to speak highly of the institutional strengths of socialism with Chinese characteristics. On May 17, the WHO convened a meeting on fighting against the pandemic. The publishing of Modrow's article in the German media gave support to China, which was of important significance. – *Li Ruiqin, Wang Jianzheng.*

1   Li Ruiqin, research fellow of the Academy of Marxism, Chinese Academy of Social Sciences.

2   Wang Jianzheng, senior advisor to China Institute for International Strategic Studies.

German Democratic Republic "joined" the Federal Republic of Germany and the GDR ceased to exist. Later, Hans Modrow became the honorary chairman of the Party of Democratic Socialism in Germany. In addition, he had been a member of the German Bundestag and the European Parliament for many years since 1994. And now he remains chairman of the Council of Elders of the Left Party.

Abstract

There is no let-up in the mainstream Western media's anti-communism ideology as COVID-19 rages throughout the world. The systematic risks pose a major challenge to the public health sector all over the world, with the results highlighting the strengths of the socialist system and the weaknesses of the capitalist system in terms of the capacity for national governance. Shouldering the "humanistic mission," China "presents to the world an image of a major country meeting its responsibilities."

I. There is no let-up in the mainstream Western media's anti-communism ideology as COVID-19 rages throughout the world

It happened at the Japanese embassy in Berlin in early 2020, when the worrisome news from China spread to Europe. In the eyes of the German politicians who were invited by the Japanese ambassador, what was happening in China was distant. Takeshi Yagi, the Japanese ambassador, warmly received his guests, and requested them to exert influences for peace and understanding in the new era. Speaking on behalf of the German guests, Volker Kauder mentioned the concept of harmony in his formal speech. Kauder is a powerful politician with considerable influences. A few weeks ago he was the leader of the ruling conservative CDU/CSU parliamentary group, a post he had assumed for 13 years. Kauder is regarded as the right-hand man of Angela Merkel, chancellor of Germany. Observers believed that Kauder's failure in getting reelected as the chairman of the parliamentary group was a result that the chancellor was losing her power. In the presence of many invited guests, Kauder adopted a measure with the significance of "tour of horizon." He blurted out the word "the Chinese pestilence (die Chinesische Seuche)."

I was shocked to hear the phrase. Having long disappeared from the German lexicon, the word "pestilence" has been replaced by a neutral word "infection (Infektion)." The word "pestilence" evokes memory of "Pest" and "Cholera," and the dark Middle Ages that existed a few centuries ago, when hygienic conditions were generally unavailable. Linking this obsolete word with China obviously reflects the speaker's contempt and anti-communism stance, and constitutes a discordant sound.

I asked a fashionably dressed lady beside me whether I had correctly understood Kauder's phrase and whether he really used the phrase of "the Chinese pestilence." The lady is a famous anchorwoman hosting the program *Journal Today* (*Heute Journal*) almost every day at the Second German Television (ZDF), which is one of the most important television stations in Germany. In my opinion, the lady has a precise mastery of the German language, and she would pay special attention to the subtle differences of words.

The lady nodded: Yes, he said so. She looked at me intently because she fully sensed the critical tone in my questions. Then she eagerly reassured me that the original intention of Kauder was by no means slander or vilification, although his remarks sounded somewhat sarcastic. She spoke in defense of Kauder, although it was not necessary to argue in favor of him at all: Kauder indeed negated Beijing and its policy (It is said the lady also used the word "the Chinese pestilence" in a television program before long. Thus "the formation of consensus" achieved its intended result.)

The experienced CDU politician displayed the self-contradictory policy of the federal government in his speech. On the one hand, Germany needs China, which serves as a market and partner of German enterprises, therefore there exists no fear of maintaining engagement with China from this perspective. The female chancellor has paid more visits to China than any other heads of the German federal government did, and she was accompanied by a horde of businessmen and representatives of combines on each of her visits to China. On the other hand, Germany is profoundly conservative about China in terms of ideology – an attitude that has always existed. The anti-communism was (and still remains) an important element of conservatism in Germany. To conservative rulers, all thoughts that are beyond the comprehension of Christianity – Western democracy are heresies without exception. In this regard, the Federal Republic of Germany unconditionally follows the US. Even when Trump was criticized for attacking China, Germany remained silent, refusing to condemn the US president. The US sets the tone as to what is fine and correct and what is evil and wrong for everything in this world. Once the criterion of "freedom and democracy" is set by the Americans, German politicians would follow it without fail.

It is because of this that it was not surprising at all for Germany to criticize China bitterly when stringent measures were adopted in Wuhan and many parts of China in early 2020. The German media were almost unanimous in their criticism: That Communist country displayed its suppressive side; people were not allowed to leave their home; they were under absolute surveillance everywhere. The German media were indignant, believing that human rights were violated. The anti-communism, which constitutes a basic element of the Federal Republic of Germany, prevents Germany from objectively analyzing the situation without reservation or without ideological bias. No matter what measures China adopts, they are all wrong – because the ruling party there is the Communist Party of China (CPC). In such a way, people lost a lot of time.

Criticism of China became much less vociferous when leaders of Europe and other countries were faced with the same challenge as the Chinese leaders did after the virus crossed national boundaries. The World Health Organization (WHO) sang praise of China for the measures it had adopted, and spoke highly of China's action of uniting with other countries and providing assistance to them. Thus, the People's

Republic of China has won praise from the international community.

The noises in criticizing China gradually died down in the Western countries. This is because Western countries have to take similar measures that China has taken earlier, not because they affirmed the actions taken by the Communist Party of China. Kindergartens, primary and secondary schools and universities are closed; theaters and museums close their doors; restaurants and bars stop operation as well; enterprises suspend production after their employees are infected by the coronavirus; the public transport is operated in a limited scale; airplanes are grounded; and national boundaries are closed...

II. The ways of responding to the epidemic highlight the strengths of the socialist system and weaknesses of the capitalist system

The public life in Europe is thoroughly paralyzed. Many people have lost the basic conditions for subsistence – including people in Germany. Small and medium-sized enterprises are in desperate conditions economically. The federal government allocated billions of euros in an effort to stop the economy from collapse. Emergency assistance, all kinds of subsidies and loans, however, can achieve short-term effects only. If the epidemic continues to spread, and the measures against the epidemic have to be prolonged beyond the expected period of time, which may result in the bankruptcy of thousands upon thousands of enterprises, what can the government do to deal with the situation? The issue has become a top priority. Mario Ohoven, president of the German Association for Small and Medium-sized Businesses (Bundesverband mittelständische Wirtschaft), gave a warning in May 2020, expressing his worry that the German enterprises hit by the COVID-19 epidemic would be purchased by Chinese investors. Then the media play the same old tune by talking about the fear of the "China threat."

In a televised speech, Chancellor Merkel stressed that the infectious disease posed the biggest political challenge since the Second World War. Cities and enterprises were almost all destroyed during the aggressive war launched by German Fascists against other countries. Millions of people became homeless vagrants wandering from one place to another in Europe. At that time, there was barely food for sustaining life, and it was almost impossible to engage in manufacturing. However, all people were equal in the sight of poverty at that time.

As things are totally different today, they cannot be compared with the situation during the wartime days. On the one hand, the wealthiest people can solve their problems with money. On the other hand, many people do not possess enough money to save life. Therefore, their lives may end up in large graves where a large number of dead people are buried. The horrible scene in New York presented the miserable condition in the city in April 2020: Bodies were laid in crude wooden coffins piled up in a long pit; then caterpillar bulldozers filled the graves with loads of earth and leveled the ground.

The misfortunes of Germany manifest themselves in another way. For instance, some people hang plastic bags full of food on the bamboo fences of the houses for the poorest of the poor, since other sources of assistance are already exhausted. The disease prevention and treatment facilities are used to their utmost capacities. Over the past decades, hospitals have been operated in the same way as enterprises. Resources that are seemingly unnecessary and redundant have been cut: manpower, sickbeds and technical apparatus. The people suffering from diseases are no longer called patients (Patienten) but are regarded as customers (Kunden) needing services. As a result, differences arise between customers purchasing personal insurance and customers covered by national statutory medical insurance. They represent the medical systems for people of two social classes, because compared with people covered by statutory medical insurance, people purchasing personal insurance can enjoy better and faster medical treatment. The current medical security is dependent upon the conditions in different localities and the market, while the responsibilities of the state are weakened.

When the number of patients contracting the infectious disease rises sharply, the weak links resulted from the resources saved in the past for for-profit purposes become all the more apparent. Sickrooms, sickbeds, manpower, technical equipment and medicines are all in short supply.

At the same time, people find to their surprise that China can complete the building of several new hospitals in just a few weeks, produce millions of face masks (It even provides face masks to other countries), and provide medical advice and assistance to other countries. WHO praises China and sets China as a good example, while the rich capitalist industrialized countries are short of medical services and supplies. These countries rapidly exceed China in both the number of confirmed cases and the number of deaths.

The virus does not discriminate on grounds of nationality or income. The difference lies in that different societies responding to the challenge in different ways. Therefore, social system becomes an issue. Such an issue has never disappeared, but nobody talks about it after the Soviet-style socialism collapsed in Europe. The Western countries are suspicious of and slander socialism with Chinese characteristics. They spare no efforts to suppress any thinking about the choice of social systems.

The outbreak of COVID-19 has made people rethink the questions that have not been discussed in public for a long time: What kind of social system is more humane? What is the position of humans among all dimensions of efforts? What social system is the one that is more in the interests of the public – Is it capitalism that regards maximization of profits as the only driving force, or is it socialism – the "society complying with the requirements for the nature of species"? The socialist system is oriented towards meeting people's real needs, rather than the needs as publicized by capitalism for meeting its profit-making purpose. The socialist system will not allow a small number of shareholders to put the surplus value of production, i.e. profits, into their own pockets; instead, it will impartially benefit everybody. What kind of political leaders will be trusted by people? – The leaders who are aware of their responsibilities for the entire society at any time and prioritize people's interests? Or the leaders who possess the lion's share of wealth of the entire country or even the entire world and make decisions based on seeking personal gains and profits for a small number of people?

The 42 richest people in the world own more wealth than 3.7 billion people, or half of the global population. Similar figures are also found in Germany: the 45 richest people possess the wealth equivalent to half of the social wealth in Germany. Will a person in his/her right mind believe that such a massive amount of wealth is obtained through decent and normal way of working?

The media here take great pains discussing the topic on systems, believing the lifestyle would surely be "different" after the infectious disease is over. It is without doubt that things will be "different," because the capitalist system not only manifests its social limit during this crisis, but also puts forward the issue on the essence of human life: The humans exist for achieving harmony in their hearts, establishing harmony with their neighbors and pursuing harmony with nature instead of engaging in production and consumption. Solidarity and mutual help are more important than being egoistic, and the spirit of solidarity and friendship is more necessary than obstinate self-imposed isolation. Only in this way can the entire society be united.

These are not fresh theories. They have been put forward by many wise men:

From Franz von Assisi to Pope Francis, the latter consciously selects this name because he believes his life's blueprint is politically practical and feasible. From Jesus to Gandhi, from Yellow Emperor to sage Albert Schweizer who traveled far to Africa and practiced medicine to help local people, from *Tao Te Ching* by Lao Tzu to *Holy Bible*, from Sakyamuni Buddha to Karl Marx, from Confucius to Xi Jinping…

Against such a backdrop, I read again the speech made by Chinese President Xi Jinping at the National Health Conference held in August 2016, which was much earlier than the outbreak of the infectious disease. In his speech, Xi Jinping pointed out the dialectical relationship between preserving health and the protection of ecological environment aimed to promote health. Protecting ecological environment means not only taking care of and protecting nature, but also caring for the special characteristics of mankind. The capitalist ways of production will ultimately lead to the extinction of humans, because they unscrupulously extort all natural resources on which human survival depends. Xi Jinping pointed out: "A good eco-environment is essential to the survival and health of mankind."[1] He believes that the understanding of "environment" should not be limited to surrounding living conditions or nature. Xi Jinping also clearly stressed the responsibility system. As the leader of the CPC and China, he pointed out, "Building a healthy China is the CPC's solemn promise to the people."[2] China should "present to the world an image of a major country meeting its responsibilities" in carrying out this "humanistic mission," and should "improve our international aid mechanism to respond to worldwide major public health emergencies, and enhance healthcare cooperation with the countries along the Belt and Road routes."[3]

III. The crisis and the decline of capitalism are inevitable following the end of the epidemic

While the epidemic in Europe gradually subsides, the symptoms of a crisis of the capitalist society are more apparent than ever. In the US, 38 million people are out of job – and the American president shifted the blame to China and its leader. In May, he claimed that China had concealed the information about the epidemic and its spread, in other words, China had cheated the entire world. His response reveals the following three points: first, it proved that Washington was incompetent and ineffective in managing domestic affairs; second, it made it clear that the US was unwilling to accept or admit that China had effectively controlled the epidemic

---

1   Xi Jinping: *The Governance of China*, Vol. II, Foreign Languages Press, 2017, p. 372.
2   Xi Jinping: *The Governance of China*, Vol. II, Foreign Languages Press, 2017, p. 373.
3   Xi Jinping: *The Governance of China*, Vol. II, Foreign Languages Press, 2017, p. 373.

and its aftermath economically, socially and politically; third, it showed that the representative of American imperialism was determined to go to the front in person and use the virus as a political weapon to attack China. As early as January 24, 2020, Trump praised China for taking tremendous efforts to bring the epidemic under control, saying that the US thought highly of China's efforts and transparency. He also expressed thanks to President Xi Jinping in the name of the American people. However, when Trump became aware that the strength of China is enhanced rather than being weakened during the crisis, he intensified the propaganda warfare with an aggressive pitch.

But the measures adopted by Trump became a boomerang that hit himself. The public mood around the world turned to be critical of the US. The German government has always been a loyal follower of the US. The pro-American sentiment in Germany was very obvious. However, a highly-reputed academic organization conducted a survey in April 2020 on Germans' views about the US and China.

In 2019, half of German people believed that the Germany-US relationship carries more weight than Germany-China relationship, while only one quarter of German people (24 percent) believed that Germany-China relationship is more important. This figure changed drastically in just one year. Although German media launched an anti-China propaganda campaign, 13 percentage points were lost in support for the US while 12 percentage points were gained in support for China. In other words, the rate of support for China (36 percent) almost leveled that for the US (37 percent). The result proves once again that people make better judgment than the government or political parties. China has received a high mark because of its good crisis management and its practical and sober-minded support for and assistance to other countries.

As an elderly politician and president of the Council of Elders of the Left Party in Germany, I search my heart to ask myself whether our party has given enough attention to these issues. The answer is no. We fail to do so from both macroscopic and microscopic perspectives. We fail to reach the height that should have been attained to rise to the present challenge in terms of theoretical thinking as well as political action – whether in Germany or within the global framework.

Any issue concerning the Left Party in Germany is in essence related to the left-wing forces in Europe. The reality that socialism is in the doldrums and the disintegration of the Soviet Union lead to not only the spiritual confusion but also the declining tendency of Marxist Thoughts, and such an effect shows no sign of ceasing. Such a phenomenon changes the actions taken by the left-wing forces when they are faced with the brutal and blood-thirsty capitalism. The force of solidarity in Europe or even Latin America is obviously at a low ebb in terms of courage, perseverance, unity and mutual help, to say nothing of the possibility of further developing Marxist Thoughts. The Left Party in Germany should not only launch social struggles in the society and in the process of globalization, and analyze and criticize the ways of shaping democracy and the ways of assuming the political leadership, but also provide tactical and strategic options. To this end, we should take the past and present experiences into consideration, including the experience being created by Chinese comrades. The Council of Elders of the Left Party will exert its influences in this respect, so that the Marxist Thoughts would be strengthened again with their prominent position restored. We need to do so immediately.

The Communist Party of China will soon hail its 100th anniversary. The Communist Party of China has lifted hundreds of millions of people out of poverty, and is still marching on this road with the goal of getting rid of poverty once and for all. Such a mission and its achievements should not only be respected but also serve as encouragement to left-wing forces in Europe to set them free from the present situation of being passively adapted to capitalist system and to proactively set a goal of building a socialist world. Our plan should include praising and respecting China's efforts in building a harmonious world.

It is becoming clearer that the founding of the People's Republic of China is a turning point in the history of the world. This is substantiated by every one of my visits to China. No difficulties – whether they are natural disasters or the coronavirus – will prevent China from marching forward on the path of development. This has been clearly proved by the objective analysis of the battle against the epidemic during the National People's Congress of the People's Republic of China held in May 2020. No matter how uproarious the propaganda against China is on the other side of the Pacific Ocean and in Europe, China has become, more than ever, the promise of the entire world.

This is why leaders in capitalist countries are anxious, and it also explains why they make a number of destructive responses that pose a threat to world peace.

Coronavirus and Capitalism

[Hungary] Thürmer Gyula

Edited by Yu Haiqing[1] Qi Jianpeng[2]

About the Author

Thürmer Gyula, born in April 1953, is a famous Hungarian politician and social activist. During the period of the People's Republic of Hungary, Gyula worked at the Ministry of Foreign Affairs and the international department of the Hungarian Socialist Workers' Party for a long time. From 1985 to 1989 he served as an advisor on diplomatic policies and security issues to Grósz Károly, the last general secretary of the Hungarian Socialist Workers' Party. After the Hungarian Socialist Workers' Party was reorganized into the Social Democratic Party of Hungary, Gyula reconstructed the Communist Party of Hungary, and renamed it Hungarian Workers' Party since Hungarian laws prohibit the use of the word "communism" in titles and logos. Since December 1989, Gyula has been chairman of the Hungarian Workers' Party.

---

1 Yu Haiqing, research fellow of the Academy of Marxism, Chinese Academy of Social Sciences.
2 Qi Jianpeng, doctoral candidate of 2018, school of Marxism, Shandong University.

Abstract

The COVID-19 epidemic has proved to be a major test for the world. China has achieved a significant victory in this test, while most of the capitalist countries are ineffective in responding to the virus. This is because the capitalist medical system following the creed of "money first" is on the brink of collapse, and the capitalist values based on profits and individualism obstruct the effective social mobilization. The epidemic exposes the crisis of capitalist integration while highlighting China's powerful governance capability and the strengths of the socialist system over capitalist system. Although capitalist countries are adopting various measures to fight the epidemic, the economic and political crises caused by the epidemic still bring many uncertainties to the world situation. To address such a situation, China proposes the concept of developing a global community of shared future, which is a realistic solution that is aimed to prevent further damages, thwart a world war, and make it possible for all countries to develop in their own ways.

Why hundreds of thousands of people have died? Why humanity cannot stop the devastation although we have all technical and scientific achievements of 21st century? The questions have been put forward by people all over the world. Coronavirus is a virus. Humanity is fighting against it. Where is it coming from? Scientists will give a clear answer. Although humanity is fighting against nature, we are living in societies and expecting social structures to help us to prevent infection and to survive the epidemic. The question is how different societies can help the struggle against the forces of nature? China has won initial victory in the fight against the epidemic and provided the whole world with valuable experiences. The epidemic has run through the European countries and the US living in capitalist societies. After two months of difficult fight against the epidemic, we can draw some conclusions about the interaction of coronavirus and capitalism.

I. Capialist Counteies responded to COVID-19 with delay

The capitalist system and the institutions of capitalism could not prevent the epidemic. But it is true that every country has been fighting against it seriously. The leading capitalist countries responded to the epidemic with delay. It can be explained by different factors:

1. The leaders of many capitalist countries considered that the developed systems of the EU countries and the USA can stop the epidemic on the borders. They neglected the warnings of the WHO and the experience of China which was published in due time. "I think that all of us are not experts and underestimate the coronavirus from the start," Ursula von der Leyen, President of the European Commission, told Germany's *Bild* newspaper in an interview.

2. Some capitalist countries realised that they could not stop the epidemic. They knew that their healthcare system is not prepared to face epidemics of such volume, but they didn't have political braveness to tell the truth to the people.

3. Capitalism is based on money and profit. Money and profit were the main factors the government took into consideration when taking concrete steps against the coronavirus. If borders would be closed too early, tourist business will lose a lot. If social isolation is introduced early, companies would have less profit. It is quite morbid, but it is true. The financial aspect was important if not dominant.

II. Capitalism: money above all

The healthcare system was one of the main players of the fight. In some countries, like Italy, France, Spain, the USA, the healthcare system collapsed practically immediately. There are different reasons connected with the main essence of capitalism. Let us see some of them!

1. Capitalist countries spend much on healthcare but not enough, The OECD (Organization for Economic Co-operation and Development) countries spend 8.8%

of the GDP. In Hungary it is 6.6%. In capitalist countries everything is expensive including doctors, assistants, medicaments, etc.

2. Privatisation of healthcare took place almost in every capitalist country. Instead of planned and proportional development of all branches of medical service only those branches which brought money were developed. This strategy undermined the basic medical services, including the regional system of local doctors. There are a lot of villages even in Hungary where the post of the doctor is vacant.

3. The healthcare system was developed with the aim that all capacities should be used as much as possible. In normal times 80%-90% percent of the capacity of the hospital was used. Capitalist countries did not have reserves for crisis time. A lot of capitalist countries reduced the number of hospital beds with the aim to rise the efficiency. In Italy there are 2.6 hospital beds/ 1000 inhabitants, in Spain 2.4, in France 3.1. When the coronavirus came there were not enough beds. Capital is interested in maximal exploitation of hospital beds. In Italy 78.9% of hospital beds are in nonstop use, While in France it is 75.6%, in Spain 75.3%. During the epidemic, the so-called intensive care beds are the most important. At the same they are the most expensive. In Spain there are 9.7 intensive beds/100 thousand inhabitants, in Italy 8.6.

4. The efficiency of the system also depends on the number of inhabitants covered by health insurance. In the USA only 35.9% of the population is covered by state insurance. 10%, i.e. 33 million Americans, does not have any insurance.

5. The accomplishment of the healthcare depends also on the system of guidance. In Italy, the whole system is decentralised where local governments decide all questions. It means there is no centralized register of hospital beds. In many countries the informatics system of the hospitals is on low level because owners did not want to invest. It is characteristic that only 0.85% of IT-specialists are engaged in healthcare.

6. Capitalist countries did not have enough workforces and material reserves.

In case of having military doctors to deal with the epidemic, medical personnel of private hospitals and pensioners can be used as extraordinary reserves. But what is the reality? In Italy with a population of 60 million, there are only 1566 military doctors, in France with a population of 66 million, there are only 1827 military doctors. Remember! At the start of the epidemic 5 thousand military medical personnel was sent to Wuhan. It became clear that the capitalist countries did not have material reserves either, for a long time there was an absolute shortage of masks, disinfectant materials etc. The hospitals had only the most necessary amount of such goods because big depots cost more. The European capitalist countries stopped the production of many medical materials because it was cheaper to produce them in developing countries. Now developed countries remained without the necessary production basis.

III. Values of capitalism did not work

The epidemic clearly demonstrates that values of capitalism is based on Profit and individualism, which disturb the society to mobilize all resources for the fight against the virus. Profit means that capitalist countries spend less on healthcare than it would be necessary. It means that private healthcare gets privilege. Individualism means that private interests are considered more important than collective interests. This principle makes exceedingly difficult to take any decision which can hurt the private interests. The political system of capitalist country based on multiparty parliaments did not allow to take the necessary decisions in due time. In many countries the problem of epidemic became a question of the fight between the government and the opposition. The moral crisis of Western capitalist societies broke the effective fight against the epidemic. The Western societies are occupied by endless discussions about human rights, gender problem, non-classical forms of sexual life. Freedom is interpreted as something absolute. There is no discipline or internal solidarity.

IV. Governance capabilities of capitalist and socialist systems

There are remarkable differences between the different European countries concerning the consequences of COVID-19. The Central and Eastern European countries are also capitalist countries but all of them are coming from socialist past.

The Central and Eastern European countries passed the COVID-19 easier than the Western countries where there has never been socialism. In Hungary for example, the healthcare system did not collapse. Socialism created a global healthcare system which is open to everybody. Although capitalists' forces have tried to destroy this system, but they could not do it fully. This system includes basic medical system of local doctors, a global system of hospitals with special epidemic hospitals included.

The governing elite of Hungary realised that a mass dissatisfaction caused by non-correct handling of COVID-19 can lead to mass demonstration against the government and even against the capitalist system generally. The government took a lot of measures to help the people. They did it not from pure humanism but with the aim to prevent any mass dissatisfaction and any action against the capitalist system. People accept all kinds of help, but they do not think about what the real intension of the capitalist government is.

These facts demonstrate that even some elements of socialism which continue existing in some Central and Eastern European countries can help the current government to face COVID-19.

China was the first country to win COVID-19. The experience of China in the fight against the epidemic is of great and global importance. The US and some other capitalist countries try to hide their own mistakes and weak points by launching attacks against China and the Communist Party of China. What were the strong points of the reaction of socialism with Chinese characteristics?

1. China could create a modern system of governance. It is accepted by the people and at the same time it is efficient. The Chinese system of governance has

demonstrated its capability. The successes of China in overcoming COVID-19 confirm the correctness of Xi Jinping Thought on Socialism with Chinese Characteristics for a New Era. The overall goal of deepening reform in every field is to improve and develop the system of socialism with Chinese characteristics and modernize China's system and capacity for governance.

It is remarkable that the Communist Party of China has launched a program of the Party and state institution reforms in early 2018. This program achieved expected results and paved the way for China's future reform measures and development. The reform has strengthened the leadership of the CPC. Central organs of the CPC have been given more management and coordination responsibilities, taking the lead in work of different areas.

China's unique governance system has shown strong vitality and huge strength. China can continuously improve itself and learn from others and is attracting more people from the international community to analyse its global significance.

2. People had full confidence in the Communist Party of China. They believed in the party which established the PRC in 1949 and led the country on the way of reform and opening after 1978. Since the outbreak of COVID-19, the CPC Central Committee has been regarding epidemic prevention and control as the top priority. The ruling Communist Party of China has achieved huge success in listening to the voice of the people, cracking down on corruption and building governance capacity. Building itself into a clean and efficient party, it can offer experience for counterparts in many other countries plagued by political chaos and deepening social divide.

3. The modern and effective system of governance could realise a rapid and effective integration of military and civil government. The reorganization of the commanding system of the Chinese armed forces was successful. Now the Chinese Supreme Command was able to concentrate large forces from different places to one place. The Chinese transport capacity has demonstrated serious development. The new China-made strategic airplanes were used in non-war action for the first

time. The Chinese system of military health care seems to have worked well. The psychological and ideological training of the Chinese soldiers and all participants of the war against the virus was on an extremely high level.

It is gratifying to note that today, due to very diligent handling of the pandemic by the medical professionals and other workers of China under the able leadership of President Xi Jinping and the Communist Party of China, the disease has come into full control in China with limited number of deaths. It is also to be noted that the Chinese workers and entire people are still taking number of extremely cautious measures to ensure the further prevention of disease in China. All these prove to show the strengths of the socialist system.

On the contrary, the countries of the capitalist world, particularly characterized by the attitude of the businessman-like president of USA, have refrained from taking necessary measures in their own countries in time and instead spent their forces in accusing China of taking so-called "inhuman measures" against the disease. After gross negligence at the beginning of disease, they are now onto the blame game against China, which is quite untenable. The capitalists looked after their petty economic interests only at the beginning and when the disease spread, they simply closed industries retrenching workers in millions of numbers. There is an unprecedented depression in capitalist economy now due to the selfish and anti-Chinese attitude of the capitalist rulers.

V. Losses and wins of capitalism

Capitalism has survived the first attack of COVID-19. Sooner or later, but all capitalist countries adopted effective measures to defeat the epidemic. People are happy to see that step by step all limitations would be cancelled and there is real hope to return to normal life. Now the economic and social consequences mean the greatest challenge.

1. Capitalism has suffered great losses because of COVID-19

Companies are suffering great losses on the stock market. In 2018 the value of the stocks of international company BOSS was 7.7 billion euro, now it is 1.7 billion. The loss is 78%. The value of the stocks of Daimler was 96.7 billion euro in 2015, now only 33.1 billion. The loss is 66%.

Air companies are losing billions every day. German air companies decreased their achievement by 90%, US companies by 74.5%. Ryanair used to have 2500 flights every day, now only 20.

The indebtedness of capitalist states is rising everywhere. The debts of Germany were on the level of 58% of the GDP in 2019, now it is 75%.

Capitalist world is facing the economic consequences of COVID-19. According to president of the European Central Bank Christine Lagarde, the GDP of the European countries would fall back by 2-10%. According to the Bloomberg, the GDP will decrease by 6%.

Europe is returning to mass unemployment. According to the McKinsey & Co, the number of unemployed will be doubled this year, achieving 7.6%. In 2021 even 11.2% is expected. In the US, 18-20% of the people are unemployed. In Turkey it is even 40%.

According to the International Labour Organization, 25 million people will be unemployed by the end of 2020. This situation will lead to enormous loss of incomes. The social consequences of the actual crisis will be remarkably like the crisis of 1929.

Traditional parties continue losing their popularity and influence. For example, the Social Democratic Party of Germany got 17% at a recent public opinion poll which is the lowest in their history.

2. What are the most important wins of capitalism because of COVID-19?

The capitalist forces will use the epidemic to realise some measures which are impossible in peace time. A lot of state money will be sent on defence, security industry, air transport and private healthcare. Inflation is attacking all capitalist countries. The rise of prices means losses for large groups of the people, but capitalist state wins a lot. As Milton Friedman said: "Inflation is taxation without legislation." The capitalist forces will try to take the societies under full control. They want to introduce the compulsory tests, the digital following of the virus, control of mobiles etc. The capitalist forces will force the working masses to pay for the crisis. We see already that governments support the banks and transnational companies. Prices are also going up and we can expect an even higher inflation.

The question is whether the actual crisis would lead to such consequences as the crisis of 1929 led, or capitalism can avoid general collapse. There is a common opinion that COVID-19 is turning into a global economic crisis. The capitalist countries and organizations try to prevent the economic crisis from becoming a global social crisis which would be able to shake capitalist order. The problem is not the economy itself. The real problem is that Europe faces different problems at the same time and most of the European societies are now weaker than in 2008. There are big differences in comparison with the crisis of 2008. First, we are facing a health crisis which concerns all countries and all social groups. Second, the migration and the reform of the EU undermined the capacities of the European structures. Third, now besides Russia, China also can influence the outcome of the crisis.

The coronavirus epidemic itself can be solved. The crisis of Europe is not connected with the coronavirus. But the epidemic will show in a more transparent way the internal problems of Europe. The European societies have lost their energy of development. The Western European societies are vulnerable. The societies are deeply divided. There are no strong leaders with force and respect.

The fear of the coronavirus resonated with the previous anti-globalism can lead to ideological self-deception.

War remains a possibility for the capitalist countries. We think that the capital will not risk a world war. They know that both world wars led to the strengthening of socialism. They do not want it. Capitalist countries are taking measures to prevent a global collapse and social revolutions. For instance:

(1) Capitalist countries and their international organizations will provide exceptional support for banks and large companies in response to the economic slowdown linked to the COVID-19 epidemic.

(2) The middle classes have lost a lot during the recent period. Capitalist governments try to stabilize their position. They will help the small and medium enterprises which are an essential driving force for capitalist societies.

(3) NATO is elaborating a security plan to safeguard the peace and security of the NATO countries.

(4) Capitalist governments work out internal political plans to defend democratic order in their countries.

VI. Collapse, devastation or building a community with a shared future for humanity

In spite of the negative consequences of COVID-19 and the economic crisis for the population, there is no revolutionary situation in any European countries now. But criticism of capitalism, attacks against the EU and the NATO are rising everywhere. There are a lot of people disappointed in capitalism.

There are a lot of uncertain moments. We do not know whether there would be a war in Europe, but we cannot exclude this possibility. The capitalist forces are fighting for new markets. The NATO and the EU try to go to the East, but they meet the ambitions of Russia. The struggle inside the EU continues. The question whether the EU would be turned into a supranational European state or the EU will be an organization of strong national states has not been decided yet. We do not know whether international capital can mobilize enough financial and other means to prevent social conflicts. But social conflicts are on the agenda in any case. We do not know either if the European communist movement can be stronger or not. As you know many parties have a lot of difficulties.

China proposes and upholds the vision of building a community with a shared future for humanity. General Secretary Xi Jinping of the Central Committee of the Communist Party of China (CPC) has put forward relevant proposals on many occasions including the Extraordinary G20 Leaders' Summit on COVID-19 and telephone conversations with other heads of state. It is a realistic way to prevent further devastations, to stop the moving to world war and to give to all nations the possibility to develop in their own way.

The world is now beset with a rising wave of anti-globalization and trade protectionism, adding uncertainty and risk to the global economy. China, now the world's largest growth engine, has been a staunch supporter of globalization and multilateral trade system.

China has been sticking to its fundamental national policy of reform and opening up, liberalizing, and facilitating trade and investment to promote an open world economy. China is committed to improving global governance, bridging the gap between the developed and developing countries and promoting a more fair and reasonable international order. The Belt and Road Initiative, an innovation endeavour proposed by China for global governance, has attracted widespread participation. The efforts not only help to meet the country's economic and social development goals and realize the great rejuvenation of the Chinese nation but are also conducive to global growth and the international multilateral system.

The COVID-19 Pandemic Marks a Turning Point in the World History

[Italy] Andrea Catone

Edited by Li Kaixuan[1]

About the Author

Andrea Catone is the editor-in-chief of *Marx Twenty-one (Marx Ventuno)*, an Italian magazine on communism, and a guest professor at the College of Marxism of Tianjin Normal University. He was born in Bari, a port city in the south of Italy in 1950, and joined the Italian Communist Youth Federation in 1966. He majored in philosophy in the university, and obtained a doctoral degree with his research on the economic-social structure of the Soviet Union. He has published many books in Italian and other languages on the Marxist theory, the Soviet Union and other socialist countries, history of workers' movement in Italy, the American politics in the post-cold war period, the invasion of imperialism and how Marxism is stigmatized. As the editor-in-chief of *Marx Ventuno* and the person-in-charge of the namesake publishing house, Andrea Catone has published several books on socialism with Chinese characteristics in Italy.

---

1   Li Kaixuan, associate research fellow of the Academy of Marxism, Chinese Academy of Social Sciences.

Abstract

The wide spread of the COVID-19 pandemic marks a turning point in the world history. It has triggered a crisis in public health, economy, politics and culture, and the ultimate way out could be either progressive or regressive. China and its president point out a progressive path: building a global community of shared future to strengthen international solidarity in the field of public health, and prioritize the health and wellbeing of people in all countries. The largest obstacle on the path of progress is "America First" preached by the American ruling class, the military industrial group behind it and American dollar – the currency of the international trade. In its response to China's collaboration initiative, the US launches a large-scale anti-Chinese campaign, and tries to harness the EU – China's largest trade partner – in this campaign. To achieve its goal, the US attempts to start a "New Cold War" based on bipolarism. However, the progressive forces and the workers' movement in the world are all working to build a multi-polarization world, with "Belt and Road" Initiative as one of its mainstays. In a more difficult and complicated new historical stage, the socialist forces in the world should fundamentally model themselves after China to promote international solidarity and cooperation and move forward on the path of building a global community of shared future.

I. Two opposing lines: The COVID-19 is a battleground between progress and reaction

It is common opinion that the pandemic, still in progress, marks a turning point in world history, so that we will talk about a world before and after COVID-19. The pandemic has opened a phase of crisis in the world, which has general characteristics common to all countries and crosses with particular characteristics of each country. As it has been for every crisis in the history of humanity, this crisis is also substantially open towards two antithetical solutions:

The first one is a progressive outlet, which will make an important step forward in the historical path of humanity, towards the realization of those ideals of freedom, equality, solidarity, omnilateral development of the human person (Marx) which were at the basis of the French Revolution of 1789 and then of the socialist revolutions of the 20th century.

The second is a regressive outlet, which will block human development for a historical phase, constitute a retreat in political, economic, social and institutions, produce greater inequality, greater poverty, greater social injustice, increasing the danger of war.

COVID-19 is a battleground between progress and reaction.

Already in the course of the development of the pandemic and its spread with unequal rhythms, times and modes in the various areas and countries of the world and the contrast to it, two opposing trends have emerged:

On the one hand, governments have taken the warnings and advice of scientists and doctors seriously, and have considered that the most effective and necessary measure – for the state reached so far by scientific knowledge on the subject – was that of rigorously blocking physical contact between people, adopting economically, as well as socially and culturally, very heavy measures to block (lockdown) activities, so as to isolate the virus and remove its fundamental basis – human beings – in which it is kept alive and reproduces. The first country – the most populous in the world – that adopted this very difficult choice was the PRC, with its very strict virus containment measures. When news of the Chinese blockade arrived at the end of January, commentators from many European countries were incredulous and astonished. There was no shortage of the usual anti-Chinese arrogance, which claimed that only a dictatorial country could implement similar measures.[1] Stopping the economic and social activities of the "factory of the world," the country that more than any other provides the world with intermediate components and finished products, was one of

---

1   See for example Pierre Haski, "La gestione autoritaria dell'epidemia di coronavirus da parte della Cina (The authoritarian management of the coronavirus epidemic by China,)" in "Internazionale," 14-2-2020, https://www.internazionale.it/opinione/pierre-haski/2020/02/18/cina-coronavirus-autoritarismo.

the most difficult decisions that the leaders of the PRC had to make. But the socialist principle that inspires the PRC has led them to put human health first, realizing that the country's economy, an economy that is also planned – albeit in a different way from Soviet planning – would suffer heavily from the blockade.

On the other hand, political leaders and governments who, in order to avoid the blockade of the economy, preferred not to listen to what the world medical science said, belittled the danger of spreading the virus, or abandoned themselves to strange theories without scientific basis, regressing from the level of modern science – which follows the Galilean method – to that of magicians, sorcerers and charlatans, presenting themselves as inventors of easy recipes to overcome the virus. The most sensational case was that of US President Donald Trump, who recommended injecting himself with varicin to kill the virus and forced all American manufacturers and sellers of disinfectants, as well as the major American TV and media, to deny and warn of the deadly danger that such advice entailed.[1] In order not to stop the economic machine of their country, the highest representatives of the major capitalist powers in the world have torn the modern scientific revolution to shreds, have regressed to charlatanism and magic, have shown in fact how much has decayed that bourgeois class that in the rise of the modern age married science and the Enlightenment as Marx and Engels write in the pages of the *Manifesto* of 1848. In good company with Trump is also the Brazilian President Jair Bolsonaro, denounced at the beginning of April by the Brazilian Association of Jurists for Democracy (ABJD) for having through his actions "substantially endanger the physical health and well-being of the Brazilian population, exposing them to a lethal virus [...] echoing unscrupulous businessmen, he has stubbornly refused to adopt the world standard of combating the pandemic, social confinement. Thus, Brazil due to the actions of President Bolsonaro ceases to participate in the strategy to flatten

---

1   See "Trump claims controversial comment about injecting disinfectants was 'sarcastic'," in *The Whashington Post*, 24-4-2020, https://www.washingtonpost.com/nation/2020/04/24/disinfectant-injection-coronavirus-trump/.

the infection curve. Rather, he seeks to expand it. Bolsonaro's conduct inevitably will cause the health system in Brazil to collapse."[1]

Although the governments of the main Western capitalist countries had had the great advantage of being able to know the experience of the Chinese bloc and its success in containing the virus – when the first outbreaks were ignited in Italy in the third decade of February, the spread of the contagion in China was almost completely blocked – they showed themselves to be rather uncertain and swinging on the blockade. The Italian government, however, after a phase of uncertainty and blockades limited to certain areas, decided to adopt the blockade in the whole country. Generally speaking, almost all European countries adopt rigid blocking measures, after a more or less long phase of uncertainty and hesitation due to the attempt to limit the economic damage of the blockade.

The countries such as Trump's USA and Bolsonaro's Brazil that have most opposed the use of the blockade of activities and the physical distance between people are today with the highest number of infectious people and deaths.

In dealing with the virus, two lines, two different conceptions of the world, have substantially manifested themselves. One, which places the value of human life first and has accepted the need to sacrifice the economy; the other, which instead places economic interest above the value of life.

II. The role of the public health system

A second aspect that divides the different countries of the world is given not only by the political choice that has oriented the decisions of closure or not, but by the health system and the overall political system of the country. The containment of contagion, in fact, is strongly influenced by the efficiency of the political system,

---

1   See "Bolsonaro denounced for crimes against humanity before the International Criminal Court," 3-4-2020, https://peoplesdispatch.org/2020/04/03/bolsonaro-denounced-for-crimes-against-humanity-before-the-international-criminal-court/.

its ability to effectively implement the decisions taken, to ensure that they are consciously implemented by the population. What is done under coercion always works much less than what is done as a conscious choice: this is what several Western commentators didn't understand about China, which has been successful in the fight against COVID-19 because its 1.4 billion people have consciously, disciplined and actively followed the indications of the CPC.

Here too the world is divided on the basis of the efficiency of the public health system. The reason for the health disaster in Lombardy – the Italian region that had the highest number of infected and deaths[1] – is to be found in the abandonment of territorial care and the privatization of the Lombardy health care: in 1981 there were 530 thousand beds in Lombardy, today there are less than 215 thousand, the local health units (USL) were 642, while in 2017 only 97. This impoverishment explains the chain of errors that led to the COVID-19 disaster. The territorial network that should have taken charge of patients has been dismantled, the emergency rooms have become places of contagion instead of prevention and the hospitals overwhelmed by the arrival of already serious patients.[2] Another element of weakness was the insufficient number of tampons, the difficulty of tracing the contagion and, therefore, an inadequate diagnostic health facility. The high number of deaths in Lombardy and in Italy as a whole lays bare the inefficiencies and deficits of Italian health care, which had one of the most advanced universal health services in the world, established with the 1978 reform, the result of the struggles conducted by the workers' movement during the decade (1968-1978) in which it was most present and active in Italian society.

---

1   Lombardy has 10 million and 84,000 inhabitants, a little less than the inhabitants of the city of Wuhan. As of May 21, according to data from the Ministry of Health (http://www.salute.gov.it/imgs/C_17_notizie_4792_0_file.pdf) there are just over 86,000 infected and 15,727 deaths.
2   See "Virus Lombardia, la crisi del modello 'Pirellone': la catena di errori che ha fatto dilagare i contagi (Virus Lombardy, the crisis of the 'Pirellone' model: the chain of errors that has spread the contagions)," "Il Messaggero," 21-5-2020, https://www.ilmessaggero.it/italia/lombardia_coronavirus_contagi_covid_19_morti_oggi_news-5242285.html.

The worst situation is in the USA, where healthcare is essentially private and aimed at capitalist profit: here the existing data reveal deep inequalities by race, especially for American blacks. As of May 19, 2020, the overall mortality rate of COVID-19 for American blacks is 2.4 times higher than for whites; in Arizona, the mortality rate for indigenous people is more than five times higher than for all other groups, while in New Mexico, the rate is seven times higher than for all other groups.[1]

It is clear that public health must be strengthened where it exists, or must be fully built. The universal right to health cannot be guaranteed by private enterprise, but only by the public sector, democratically directed and governed by representatives of the citizens. It is essential to expand the investment of public resources in the health and pharmaceutical system and equipment (in everything related to health). The capitalist system cannot effectively cure pandemics, because the investments and research of multinationals are motivated by the tension for maximum profit and not by the health of the popular masses.[2] A country oriented towards socialism like the PRC, on the contrary, will have no difficulty in further strengthening the health system in the name of the priority of human health.

The way in which a reform and strengthening of the public health service, which considers health as a universal right of the entire population, will be undertaken in the various countries will mark a clear dividing line between the two possible outlets for the crisis. The COVID-19 pandemic has found several countries unprepared. If humanity is not blind, it knows that this pandemic will not be the last and that lessons must be learned. It means strengthening prevention and territorial medicine, diagnostic systems and investing in research.

---

1   See "The color of coronavirus: COVID-19 deaths by race and ethnicity in the U.S," https://www. apmresearchlab.org/covid/deaths-by-race.

2   A recent article by Prabir Purkayastha, founder and editor-in-chief of Newsclick: "Why Capitalism Can't Cure Global Pandemics?", https://citizentruth.org/why-capitalism-cant-cure-global-pandemics/, makes this clear and timely.

III. Facing the pandemic: international cooperation or "America first"?

This pandemic has also shown that strong international cooperation is needed, conceiving the universal right to health for all humanity on all five continents. Here too, two opposing lines have emerged:

On the one hand, the tendency to strengthen not only the health system and research in individual countries, but to cooperate in research and production of mass drugs, vaccines, worldwide; then, the strengthening of the WHO, the sharing of research and medical-scientific knowledge around the world, the building of a shared future community for health worldwide. This proposal was made by Xi Jinping at the G20 on March 26, 2020, "Major infectious disease is the enemy of all [...] At such a moment, it is imperative for the international community to strengthen confidence, act with unity and "work together in a collective response. We must comprehensively step up international cooperation and foster greater synergy so that humanity" as one could win the battle against such a major infectious disease. [...] I propose that a G20 health ministers' meeting be convened as quick as possible to improve information sharing, strengthen cooperation on drugs, vaccines and epidemic control, and cut off cross-border infections. G20 members need to jointly help developing countries with weak public health systems enhance preparedness and response. [...] Guided by the vision of building a community with a shared future for mankind, China will be more than ready to share our good practices, conduct joint research and development of drugs and vaccines, and provide assistance where we can to countries hit by the growing outbreak. [...] It is imperative that countries pool their strengths and speed up research and development of drugs, vaccines and testing capabilities in the hope to achieve early breakthrough to the benefit of all."[1]

And again, at the World Health Assembly on May 18, 2020, "We must always put the people first, for nothing in the world is more precious than people's lives. [...] We need to step up information sharing, exchange experience and best practice, and pursue international cooperation on testing methods, clinical treatment, and vaccine and medicine research and development. [...] China calls on the international community to increase political and financial support for WHO so as to mobilize resources worldwide to defeat the virus. [...] We must provide greater support for Africa. Developing countries, African countries in particular, have weaker public health systems. Helping them build capacity must be our top priority in the COVID-19 response. [...] We must strengthen global governance in the area of public health. [...] In view of the weaknesses and deficiencies exposed by COVID-19, we need to improve the governance system for public health security. We need to respond more quickly to public health emergencies and establish global and regional reserve centers of anti-epidemic supplies [...] we must strengthen international cooperation. Mankind is a community with a shared future. Solidarity and cooperation is our most powerful weapon for defeating the virus."[2]

The Chinese president starts from a universalistic conception: he considers the well-being of humanity as a common good, beyond the borders and systems of states. It is a simple, common sense and at the same time great proposal: sharing knowledge, cooperating in the research of drugs and vaccines, fostering the birth of a world health system, creating networks of research and world production of drugs and health equipment, helping the less advanced countries. So, there are no patents, no properties on vaccines and medicines against epidemics.

---

1 See "Full text of Xi's remarks at Extraordinary G20 Leaders' summit," source: *Xinhua* 2020-03-26, http://www.xinhuanet.com/english/2020-03/26/c_138920685.htm. The italics in Xi Jinping's text are mine, A.C.

2 See "Full text: Speech by President Xi Jinping at opening of 73rd World Health Assembly," http://www.xinhuanet.com/english/2020-05/18/c_139067018.htm. The italics in Xi Jinping's text are mine, A.C.

This universalistic and progressive conception, in the direction of the unification of the human race, exposed by Xi Jinping, is contrasted by a narrow and petty vision of medical-scientific research and health as a private monopoly, for profit or for the exclusive benefit of one country to the detriment of others. Donald Trump fully represents this regressive trend, as he has shown on more than one occasion, seeking exclusivity on vaccines. He tried first with the German biopharmaceutical company CureVac, then with the French pharmaceutical group Sanofi. And he repeatedly attacks the WHO, accused of "alarming lack of independence from the People's Republic of China," announcing the suspension of US funding to the organization (on April 14, 2020) and threatening with an ultimatum on May 18 to cut it definitively "if the World Health Organization does not commit to major substantive improvements within the next 30 days" in order to "demonstrate independence from China." It is illuminating and revealing of the conception that has D. Trump of the international bodies the conclusion of his letter, "I cannot allow American taxpayer dollars to continue to finance an organization that, in its present state, is so clearly not serving America's interests."

Thus, the highest representative of world imperialism, the one who continually affirms "America first," the USA first and above all else, cannot anywhere near conceive of the possibility of cooperation aimed at safeguarding the health of all human beings and not just the Americans (who, by the way, with his disastrous conduct of the COVID-19 emergency, sentenced more people to death than any other country in the world). The political conception and practice of the absolute primacy of the United States, which belongs to the entire American ruling classand not only to Trumpis the main obstacle to the path of emancipation and progress of the peoples of the world and the main threat to peace.

IV. With the pandemic, the US attack on China does not retreat, but intensifies.

As the pandemic began to spread exponentially in the USA in the third week of March (on March 27, 2020, the number of contagions, over 100 thousand, exceeded those in the PRC), one might have expected that the Chinese President's call for international health cooperation, expressed clearly and distinctly at the G20 on March 26, would be accepted by the US President; but this was not the case. On the contrary, we are witnessing a crescendo of harder and harder attacks on the PRC, of which, as we write these notes, we cannot see the end.

After the first attacks on the WHO, accused of being "China-centric," on April 17, 2020, the National Republican Senatorial Committee published the *Corona big book*, a 57-page guide for Republican candidates, which indicates as the focus of the election campaign the attack on the PRC and the CPC: a real anti-Chinese booklet that prescribes three main lines of aggression: a) China caused the virus "covering it"; b) Republicans will push for sanctions against China for its role in the spread of this pandemic; c) Democrats are "soft on China."

Between April and May 2020, the anti-Chinese campaign is deployed at full speed by every means, not only in the USA, but in all the countries in the world where US-controlled media can reach. One of the weapons that in this mad campaign the American administration uses abundantly is that of legal action to obtain from the PRC, accused of "being responsible for the propagation of the virus," "billionaire reparations." "Legal" action considered by many jurists to be absurd and destined for nothing, but with a considerable propaganda impact, aimed at creating a climate unfavourable to China, put on the bench of the accused. On April 27, Trump announced a very serious claim for "damages." Trump Counsellor George Sorial, a former Trump Organization executive, brings a class action for "damages" against Beijing in the United States. Some influential media and even consumer associations are moving in different countries announcing similar claims.

On April 16, the most popular German daily newspaper, *Bild*, does so clamorously, claiming 162 billion dollars in "compensation" from China. A few days later, the Italian Coordination of Associations for the Protection of the Environment and Consumer Rights (Codacons) takes up arms and luggage alongside the Trump's anti-Chinese campaign; on April 23, its website opens with the invitation: "Book to join free of charge the Codacons action for damages against China, for the serious responsibilities and omissions in the fight against the spread of the COVID-19"; the action is carried out in collaboration with the American law firm Kenneth B. Moll. On April 29, the President of the Lombardy region, Attilio Fontana, also announced a claim for "compensation" of 20 billion euros.

On April 29, Trump, following the old French proverb "calomniez, calomniez, il en restera toujours quelque chose," for which a constantly repeated lie will end up appearing as truth, accentuates the campaign of attacks and slander against China, without providing any explanation, let alone proof.

In an even more aggressive and battling manner, fuelling a climate in which there is more and more air of war on all sides, the Trump entourage moves: someone proposes to ask China 10 million dollars for each US victim of the virus, with the aim, indicated by Trump himself, to snatch hundreds of billions of dollars from China; Republican Senator Marsha Blackburn argues that "China has cost the US economy six thousand billion and could cost another five thousand" and proposes to get compensation by no longer paying China interest on the US Treasury bonds that it owns. Others think of new trade tariffs. Or the imposition of sanctions worth a trillion dollars on future Chinese imports.[1] On May 1, a report by the US Department of Homeland Security, shared with law enforcement and government agencies, goes even higher, accusing the Chinese government of intentionally hiding severity of coronavirus epidemic while stockpiling supplies:

---

1   Marco Valsania, "Trump, Tutte le Idee per una Rappresaglia contro la Cina," May 1, 2020, see https://www.ilsole24ore.com/art/trump-tutte-idee-una-rappresaglia-contro-cina-ADp9gsN.

"the Chinese government intentionally concealed the severity of COVID-19 from the international community in early January while it stockpiled medical supplies by both increasing imports and decreasing exports. [...] China likely cut its exports of medical supplies prior to its January WHO notification that COVID-19 is a contagion."[1] As you can see, everything is being done to present the PRC and the CPC in the worst light.

The US leaders, Republican or Democrat, are used to slandering their enemies in front of the world and impudently exhibiting "evidence" that does not exist. Suffice it to recall here the vial full of white powder agitated by the then Secretary of State Colin Powell at the UN Security Council on February 5, 2003 to accuse Iraq of producing chemical and bacteriological weapons of mass destruction which, after the Anglo-American occupation of the country, continually sought, turned out to be non-existent.

At the beginning of May, the US administration cut the investment links between the US federal pension funds and Chinese shares to a value of about 4 billion dollars, claiming that this would involve investment risks and national security. On May 14, in an interview with "FOX Business" Trump threatened to sever all trade and economic relations with the PRC, claiming that this would save the US $500 billion.

Added to all this are the recent positions taken by the US administration towards Taiwan province, which, treating the island as de facto "independent," tend to disregard the principle of one China (the People's Republic of China), established since 1992 and recognized in hundreds of international agreements. Lucio Caracciolo, Editor in Chief of the Italian geopolitical magazine *Limes*, writes on this subject in his editorial of May 25:

Recent cases confirm that Washington has taken off its gloves to beat hard.

---

1   See "US intel believes China hid severity of coronavirus epidemic while stockpiling supplies," "ABC" 3-5-2020, https://abcnews.go.com/US/coronavirus-live-updates-us-surpasses-65000-covid-19/story?id=70467380.

With protocol semantics, when Secretary of State Pompeo congratulates Tsai Ing-Wen, re-elected to the presidency of the "Republic of China (Taiwan)," calling her "President," i.e. Head of State. With the violence of economic reprisal, announcing that Taiwan Seminconductor Manufacturing (world leader) will open a factory in Arizona, while banning the sale of its semiconductors in Beijing. Huawei and his 5G are under attack.[1]

Equally aggressive is the US administration's stance on Hong Kong SAR, where it foments and supports secessionist and anti-communist movements and now mobilizes its media apparatus to attack the Chinese National People's Congress to draft a national security law for Hong Kong SAR.

At the same time, the US is stepping up its military action in the seas of China. The *South China Morning Post* of May 10, 2020 writes:

So far this year, aircraft from the US armed forces have conducted 39 flights over the South China Sea, East China Sea, Yellow Sea and the Taiwan Strait – more than three times the number carried out in the equivalent period of 2019. [...] Meanwhile, the US Navy conducted four freedom of navigation operations in the South China Sea in the first four months of the year – compared with just eight for the whole of 2019 – with the latest on April 29, 2020 as guided-missile cruiser *USS Bunker Hill* sailed through the Spratly Islands chain.[2]

V. The US attack on PRC: contingent or structural?

In the face of this avalanche of increasingly warlike official statements, accompanied by political, legal, economic and military hostilities all over the world,

1   Lucio Caracciolo, "Taiwan è il Grimaldello con cui gli Usa Vogliono Scardinare la Cina," May 25,2020, see https://www.limesonline.com/rubrica/taiwan-usa-cina-indipendenza-lucio-caracciolo-editoriale.
2   Kristin Huang, "US-China tensions in South China Sea fuelled by increase in military operations," May 10, 2020, https://www.scmp.com/news/china/military/article/3083698/us-china-tensions-south-china-sea-fuelled-increase-military.

the question arises as to whether this is a temporary, contingent situation, essentially linked, on the one hand, to the attempt to hijack against China, on the other hand, to the presidential election campaign on November 2020, as the *Corona big book*, the instruction manual for Republican candidates, would seem to suggest. Several observers and political commentators have insisted on this contingent aspect, linked to the capture of the internal US consensus. It is likely that Trump's need to make up lost ground in the US electorate has contributed to inflaming the tone of the most demagogic president in US history and to increase the clash with China. His rival, Democrat Joe Biden, is doing better in his voting intentions than Hillary Clinton in 2016; a survey by *Fox News* (Trump's "friendliest" TV), confirmed by an average of the polls of the week 18-24 May, gives the Democratic candidate at 48% and the incumbent president at 40%.[1]

However, there is more than one reason to believe that the current violent US attack against the PRC is not temporary and occasional, but rather structural, rooted in the economic-political system of the United States, in the fundamental traits of the dominant class, which, democratic or republican, shares the ideology of "America first," of the US primacy in the world, of US unipolarity which does not accept and cannot be reconciled with the prospect of a multipolar world.

The USA is not and does not conceive of itself as a capitalist country like the others, nor as a "primus inter pares." The ideology of the absolute primacy of the United States was forged during the "Cold War" (1946-1991) and was openly proclaimed in the White House's strategic documents in the aftermath of the dissolution of the Union of Soviet Socialist Republics (USSR); in them the will to maintain and strengthen US unipolarism is affirmed. This unipolarity has a strong anchorage in the military-industrial complex, which expanded enormously with the

---

1   See the survey published on 21 April 2020 by the PEW Research Center: https://www.pewresearch.org/global/2020/04/21/u-s-views-of-china-increasingly-negative-amid-coronavirus-outbreak/; see also https://www.agi.it/estero/news/2020-04-21/cina-usa-sondaggio-8399936/; and https://www.agi.it/estero/news/2020-05-24/sondaggi-trump-biden-usa-2020-8711919/.

Second World War and even more so with the "Cold War."

The "Cold War," the permanent confrontation with the USSR and the "socialist camp," designated as the absolute enemy, the "empire of evil," the perennial threat to the freedom and values of the West, served the US ruling class to a) compact under its own military, political, economic command the capitalist countries of Europe and Asia (while Latin America was the "backyard" of Uncle Sam); b) to feed and extend an enormous military-industrial complex that has no equal in the world (US military spending in 2019 was 732 billion dollars);[1] c) to impose the dollar as a currency for international trade; d) to inoculate in the US population a nationalism of great power that needs to continuously feed on a great enemy, a great and threatening evil against which to fight, presenting itself as a super empire of good.

The ruling class in the USA is the centre, the beating heart of the world imperialist system and has become too accustomed to enjoying the privileges that this centrality gives it. The possible loss of world supremacy alarms the US economic potentates, who can maintain a world role by leveraging the political-military power of the country. This primacy is not only military, political, economic, it is also ideological-cultural, in soft power, and colonizes the imagination of the world population. Losing this primacy is today the main concern of the US ruling class, which sees the branch on which it sits sawed off.

This peculiar US structure can explain the violent attack on China. The US ruling class has built consensus on the American primacy in the world, and on the fight against the enemy. The American mentality, starting from World War II, and even more from the outbreak of the "Cold War," was built on the perennial image of a dark enemy: from World War II, when the enemy was the Japanese and the German Nazis, to the "Cold War" when the Communists and the USSR were the

---

1   See Manlio Dinucci, "La pandemia della spesa militare (The military spending pandemic)," in *il manifesto*, 5 maggio 2020, https://ilmanifesto.it/la-pandemia-della-spesa-militare/.

enemy, to the post-cold war when Islamist terrorism was one phase, and finally China. In order to keep the internal cohesion Trump, and not only he, but the entire American ruling class, must find an enemy, and refusing to find it in itself and in its economic-social structure, hurls himself against China.

The "election" of PRC as an enemy *par excellence* is not by chance, nor is it only contingent. It was already present between the lines in the strategic doctrine of the USA in the 1990s. And it became the obsession of the American dominant class – bipartisan, crossing both the Republican and Democratic parties – after the great financial crisis of 2007-2008. Also the PRC suffered the repercussions of that crisis, but – thanks to the socialist oriented system, to the effective capacity of the CPC to orient and direct the economy – it was able to reorganize itself rapidly, continuing with excellent performance, becoming in 2010 the second world economy and continuing on its path of internal development, of progressive overcoming of the bands of poverty present in the country, of creating the largest domestic market. Its political system, moreover, strengthened and increased social cohesion; the CPC proposed at the 19th Congress (2017) to solve the new contradictions that the development of the previous years had created, and set itself as a country that – unique in the world – spoke to the whole world proposing, contrary to the imperialist globalization of the USA, a shared path of win-win development in a multipolar world, of which the great project of the New Silk Road is a fundamental pillar.

Trump's presidency has been characterized – making the tare of some oscillations and statements that theatrically distinguish this personage – by placing China as an adversary, and then main enemy, against which he started a hard trade war in 2017. This war, even if in a zig-zag path, was in crescendo, caused great unrest in world markets and basically started a backwards path in globalization and international production chains. The three years of the Trump presidency preceding the COVID-19 pandemic have seen a gradual increase in economic attacks on China, but that is not all. Anti-Chinese media propaganda has intensified, the USA has fomented anti-Chinese movements in Hong Kong, China, has spread lies about the "repression of the Uighurs," in short, as they had well learned to do in the period of the "Cold War," when US President Ronald Reagan called the USSR "empire of evil."

VI. Europe theatre of Trump's attack on China

That the growing number of attacks on China has a base that goes well beyond the election campaign, also shows us the great media mobilisation and strong political pressure – a real "let's tighten ranks!" – of the USA towards countries linked to them by military or commercial treaties, with the clear objective of aligning them against Beijing. These are countries which, although with economic-political systems very different from that of the PRC, have developed commercial and cultural relations with it over the last few decades.

One of the most relevant areas of the world – if not the main one – on which the policy of the United States is aiming to align it with the anti-Chinese attack is Europe (understood not as geographical Europe, therefore, Russia excluded). China is the EU's second largest trading partner after the US and the EU is China's first trading partner.[1] Both sides are committed to a comprehensive strategic partnership, as expressed in the *Strategic Agenda for EU-China Cooperation 2020*. There is also the 17+1 cooperation of Central and Eastern European Countries (CEECs) for the Belt and Road Initiative.[2] In spring 2019 the main Western European countries

---

1   In 2017, the EU was China's main partner, with 13% of goods exports to China (€217 billion) and 16% of goods imports from China (€332 billion). In the same year, China accounted for 11% of exports of non-EU goods (€198 billion) and was the largest trading partner, with 20% of imports of non-EU goods (€375 billion).

2   Founded in 2012 between China and sixteen Central and Eastern European countries, joined by Greece (12 EU countries: Greece, Slovenia, Croatia, Czech Republic, Slovakia, Poland, Bulgaria, Romania, Hungary, Estonia, Latvia, Lithuania and five non-EU countries: Albania, Bosnia and Herzegovina, Montenegro, North Macedonia, Serbia), it was born as an initiative of the Chinese government to promote trade relations and investment, within the Chinese Belt and Road Initiative.

signed important agreements with the PRC on the New Silk Road, emphasized by the visit of President Xi Jinping. Italy, the first G7 country, signed the *Memorandum of Understanding*.

During the pandemic China lent considerable aid to Italy and a survey in March 2020 indicated that the PRC was considered a friendly country by the majority of Italians.[1] The political forces of the present government – although with some differences – look to China with prospects of economic collaboration and growth of interchange, including cultural exchange. For some of them, collaboration with China could be a considerable support to face the economic crisis that has been weighing on the country for years.

The US media offensive to embark and harness European countries in the anti-Chinese crusade takes place across the board, with an abundance of means and interventions in the major media. If we look at what is today the most important European country, Germany, we can see the virulence of the anti-Chinese campaign.

Let's look at the open letter to Xi Jinping that Julian Reichelt, editor in chief of *Bild*, the best-selling newspaper in Europe (over one and a half million copies) of the Springer publishing group, published in mid-April. The newspaper had become a spokesman for the campaign orchestrated by Washington to demand billions in compensation from China for the damage caused by the pandemic. The Chinese embassy in Berlin had addressed an open letter to *Bild* underlining the absurdity and groundlessness of this request. Reichelt wrote a very rhetorical, heavy-handed letter that was openly offensive to the PRC and Xi Jinping. What arguments does he use? He repeats the refrain on the lack of democracy, on the authoritarian, "non-transparent" regime, which "rules by surveillance" and "is a denial of freedom"; moreover, the PRC is accused of "intellectual property theft," enriching itself "with the inventions of others, instead of inventing itself"; it credits Washington's

---

1 In a survey presented at the beginning of April by SWG, 52% of those interviewed consider China a friendly country, while only 17% consider the USA as a friend. See https://formiche. net/2020/04/italiani-preferiscono-cina-usa-ue/.

unsubstantiated accusation, so it has to pay dearly; and finally, also the gift of face masks is "imperialism hidden behind a smile – a Trojan Horse." Nothing new under the sun. Reichelt vomits against China the usual clichés. Among them the "accusation" of theft of intellectual property to a country that has become – thanks to the policy of strong investments in schools and universities and in research and development – a leader in information and digital technologies (think about 5G), rather reveals the hostility, induced by the USA, to the collaboration with China for 5G.

But this rough and offensive letter pales in the face of the intervention of Mathias Döpfner, CEO of Springer, the largest German publisher. The US is calling for all the media in the anti-Chinese campaign because of the economic and political future. Germany is invited, and so are all European countries, to "decouple" with China, to give up their trade with it. Döpfner puts forward a question: "Where does Europe stand? On the side of the US or China?" And he takes up the clichés about the undemocratic, authoritarian country, etc., inviting mistrust of its "seemingly friendly and peaceful international expansion." He states that China's admission to the WTO in 2001 was "perhaps the biggest mistake made in recent history by the western market economies," since then, "the US's share in the gross world product (GWP) dropped from 20.18% in 2001 to 15.03% (2019). Europe's share dropped from 23.5% to 16.05%, a drop of 7.45% in less than two decades. While China's share increased from 7.84% to 19.24% in the same period, with an average annual growth rate of around 9%." According to Döpfner, this is due not to the intrinsic strength of China's socialist system, which combines plan and market, state-owned enterprises and private enterprises to implement long-term strategic development programs, which have made it possible to reduce poverty enormously and rapidly increase workers' wages and significantly improve their living conditions, but to "a non-democratic state capitalism that exploits easier trading and competitive conditions without subjecting itself to the same rules. Asymmetry instead of reciprocity was the result." So, says Döpfner, the US policy of "decoupling from

China" must be followed. "China or the US. It is no longer possible to go with both. [...] If Germany decides to expand its 5G infrastructure with Huawei, that will place an enormous strain on transatlantic relations. It would be a turning point, as America could no longer trust Germany." And Germany cannot and must not disassociate itself from the US, which, after its hard opposition to the USSR and the GDR, "directly and indirectly made German reunification possible." We must not allow – continues Döpfner – "the state capitalism of a totalitarian global power to continue to infiltrate or even take over key industries like banking (Deutsche Bank), automotive (Daimler, Volvo), robotics (Kuka) and trading hubs (Port of Piraeus)." Therefore, he invites Europe to continue "the traditional transatlantic alliance despite Trump, including the explicit and closer involvement of a post-Brexit UK and other allies such as Canada, Australia, Switzerland and the democratic countries of Asia" and to pursue, Germany in the first place, that is Europe's economic engine, "a strict process of decoupling from China," because "the economic ties are always political ties as well" and "we might all wake up one day to find ourselves in a gruesome society, on the side of China and the states loosely associated with it – like Russia, Iran and other autocracies." Germany, which has an annual trade volume with China of about 200 billion euros, compared to all German trade valued at 2.4 trillion euros, would suffer a heavy blow with the loss of Chinese trade, "but not insupportable."[1]

It is a very strong solicitation, coming from the main chain of newspapers in Germany, to join without ifs and buts the western camp led by the USA, which means first of all a strengthening of the link between Germany and the USA, despite some "tantrums" by Trump, and the strengthening of NATO. In this regard, there are significant political forces in Germany such as the SPD (and Die Linke) – the German Social Democratic camp – that would like to loosen the ties with the US and NATO.

---

1   Mathias Döpfner, "The coronavirus pandemic makes it clear: Europe must decide between the US and China," in *Businessinsider*, May 3, 2020, in https://www.businessinsider.com/coronavirus-pandemic-crisis-clear-europe-must-choose-us-china-2020-5?IR=T.

At the beginning of May 2020, Rolf Mützenich, the leader of the Social Democrats (SPD) in the Bundestag, called for Germany not to support US nuclear warheads. And he immediately received a harsh rebuke from the American ambassador in Berlin, Richard Grenell, who – and this is interesting to note – included among the reasons for the need to strengthen the Atlantic alliance, along with the "traditional" Russian enemy and the PRC: "The Russian invasion of Ukraine, the deployment of new nuclear-weapon-capable missiles by Russia on the periphery of Europe and new capabilities of China, North Korea and other countries make it clear that the threat is all too present."[1]

In short, there is growing American pressure for a "close ranks" of European allies. The role of NATO is now fully recovered in view of the anti-Chinese crusade. If during the election campaign and at the beginning of his term of office Trump had expressed, in his usual theatrical style, reservations about NATO's role and usefulness – but in reality he aimed rather to ask the Europeans to double their economic contribution to the Alliance – NATO is now fully defended and accredited, facing the imminent "threat" from Russia and China.

Beyond and more than Germany, where the USA is very much involved in stopping the autonomist attempts of a part of the SPD (party that governs in coalition with the CDU), there is another country in Europe that must be kept under close surveillance, Italy. This country, despite the official pro-Atlantic statements of the Defence Ministers Difesa Guerini (PD) and the Foreign minister Luiqi Di Maio (5-star Movement), manifests in the latest polls feelings of friendship towards the PRC much more than towards the USA. The order that comes from across the Atlantic and to which almost all the major media adapt is unequivocal: to demolish at all costs the image of China, and reinforce NATO against the Chinese threat. The arguments and the way they are presented are essentially similar to those used in

---

1   "Trump Envoy Accuses Germany of Undermining NATO's Nuclear Deterrent," in *Reuters-NYTimes*, May 14, 2020, https://www.nytimes.com/reuters/2020/05/14/world/europe/14reuters-germany-usa-nato.html.

Germany by Reichelt and Döpfner.

On May 4, 2020, the newspaper *La Stampa*, hosts Mark Esper, US Secretary of Defence, interviewed by Paolo Mastrolilli: "Russia and China are both taking advantage of a unique situation to advance their own interests. [...] Huawei and 5G is a prime example of this malign activity by China. This could harm our alliance. Reliance on Chinese 5G vendors, for example, could render our partners' critical systems vulnerable to disruption, manipulation, and espionage. It could also jeopardize our communication and intelligence sharing capabilities. To counter this, we are encouraging allied and U.S. tech companies to develop alternative 5G solutions."

On May 13, the newspaper *La Repubblica*, in turn, hosts an interview of the journalist Alberto D'Argenio to the Secretary General of NATO, already significant under the title: "Stoltenberg: NATO united against Russian and Chinese disinformation."[1] Russia and China, through disinformation[2] on the COVID-19, would carry out destabilizing acts against Western democracies in order to gain political influence on NATO and European Union partners. Like Esper, Stoltenberg also raises the alarm on Huawei's 5G: "Allies should avoid foreign investment that could compromise the confidentiality of our communications." NATO is thus fully enlisted in the anti-Chinese crusade.

The attack on China is carried out almost daily by the major media and right-wing exponents, acting as a sounding board for Trump and Pompeo's statements. Matteo Salvini, leader of the League (which was the first Italian party in the European elections on May 26, 2019, with 34.26% of the votes), said in the Senate, "We will join the request at least for a Commission of Inquiry to understand who

---

1 ALBERTO D'ARGENIO, "Stoltenberg: la Nato Unita contro la Disinformazione Russa e Cinese," May 13, 2020, see https://rep.repubblica.it/pwa/intervista/2020/05/13/news/stoltenberg_con_il_virus_russia_e_cina_vogliono_destabilizzare_l_occidente_-256546000/.
2 An Apulian proverb reads: "the ox says cuckold to the ass," to indicate the overthrow of the parts, where the accused liar accuses his opponent of lying. So the USA, who put out the fake new virus that escaped Wuhan's laboratory, accuse China of "disinformation."

has done and who has not done what, because we could end 2020 with the absurdity of having a single growing world economy, which is the Chinese economy which, after having voluntarily or involuntarily, it is not for me to judge it, caused a global pandemic, on the rubble of this pandemic goes to buy companies, data, telephony and hotels in Italy and around the world.[1]

He also calls, in full agreement with Trump, to reconsider the contributions of the Italian Republic to the World Health Organisation. It has already been said about the request to China for billions in compensation proposed by the President of Lombardy.

But the attack on China is also conducted in an indirect and more devious way. *Report* – the investigation broadcast by Rai3 (the "left-wing" channel of Italian Radio and Television), conducted by journalist Sigfrido Ranucci – is in line with the mainstream that tends to cast a sinister light on China. The May 11 broadcast is dedicated to an investigation into the WHO, just a few days before its 73rd World Assembly on May 18-19, at which Trump sends a letter to its Director General, accusing the WHO of being enslaved to China. *Report* fully supports this thesis.

The first part of the broadcast is dedicated to the demolition of the figure of WHO General Director Tedros Adhanom Ghebreyesus, who is shown in the broadcast sitting next to Chinese President Xi Jinping in the Great Hall of the People of Beijing (January 28). His grave guilt? To openly praise the Chinese government for the management of COVID-19, "but" – the journalist tells us – "we do not know on what basis since the WHO has not yet made a real inspection in China." But who is Tedros? Here is the evil portrait that makes the broadcast: "In his country, Ethiopia, he was minister first of Health, then of Foreign Affairs in governments that did not hesitate to use violence against the opposition. His party is the dreaded TPLF (the Popular Front for the Liberation of the Tigris) [...] During

---

1   "Salvini, Commissione Inchiesta su Cina," May 27, 2020, see https://www.ansa.it/sito/notizie/topnews/2020/05/27/salvini-commissione-inchiesta-su-cina_49085fcc-ba96-49eb-8ac1-6ffe040bba70.html.

the management of the Ethiopian government, the TPLF has been accused of many episodes of corruption. Tedros was not only a member of that government, but also a leading figure in the TPLF party. The TPLF was the main force in government."

We would therefore be dealing with a shady figure, a leading figure of a corrupt government (many episodes of corruption) and despotic (he used violence against the opposition). But that's not enough, the main force of government, the TPLF, "is linked by a double thread to the Chinese Communist Party and in particular to the figure of the current President Xi Jinping because of his heavy investments in the Ethiopian country." *Report* tells us quite explicitly that the appointment of the "first African who manages to climb to the top of the WHO" is not due to personal merit, but to China, which, thanks to the large investments in infrastructure, can influence the African Union and get him elected.

Report makes a digression on Chinese policy in Africa. Many countries on the continent – it is said with great regret – have become very attached from an economic point of view to China. But, it is also said, "this Chinese embrace of the continent was not free," but to "hold" the countries of the continent. But it's not enough: not only do the Chinese evildoers buy the director of the WHO, presented as a puppet in their hands, but they spy on the work of the Union of African Countries: "The data that passed through the headquarters of the African Union were intercepted by the Chinese government within this same structure." And here is the conclusion, the portrait of a real criminal association – Money and investment is the thread that keeps Tedros tied to China at this moment. Even the African Union would thus be a puppet in Chinese hands. This statement is dropped there, as if it were proven truth, without the "investigative journalist" bringing any evidence.

But it is still not enough, last but not least, there is an interview with Andrea Sing-Ying Lee, presented as "Taiwanese Ambassador to Italy," pretending to ignore – but they are professional journalists! – that the only Chinese Embassy in Italy is that of the PRC and that Italy, like other countries in the world, has for years adhered to the "One China" principle, a policy that now the US administration, in its mad policy of attack on the PRC, aims to overturn.

VII. "Cold War," bipolarism, unipolarism, multipolarism

The expression "New Cold War" is increasingly used in political interventions and in the media to designate the current situation of relations between the USA and the PRC. This expression – as language scholars teach us – is neither neutral nor innocent, it communicates a certain point of view to readers or listeners and tends to give a certain vision of things.

In the current language of journalism, but also of historians, the expression "Cold War" is used throughout the post-1945 period (end of World War II) until the demolition of the socialist countries of Central Eastern and Balkan Europe (1989) and the USSR (1991). Which configuration of world relations implied the Cold War? Basically a bipolar world, in which two great antagonistic and irreconcilable blocs, socialism and capitalism, East and West, two – so it was said – "superpowers," were confronted.

The bipolar opposition was not a choice of the Soviet leadership, but was imposed by the USA and the United Kingdom, who thus managed to align all the countries of Western Europe under the political, economic and military command of the USA. The founding of NATO in 1949 and its subsequent enlargements sealed this alignment. The Warsaw Pact only took shape several years later and was dissolved in 1991.

The concept of "West," "Western values," "Western bloc," as we still use it today, as a synonym of market economy, liberal-democracy and pro-Atlantism, also took shape after World War II in contrast to the USSR and the People's Republic of China, depicted by the West as dictatorships and barbarism. In this way, Marx and Engels, the communist thought, as well as all thought of anti-colonial and anti-imperialist emancipation, were expelled from the West.

The binary simplification of the bipolar world played in favour of the dominant class of US imperialism, which forced other countries to take sides for or against the Western bloc, excluding the possibility of intermediate and diversified positions. The birth of the movement of non-aligned countries, which we can date back to the Bandung Conference in 1955, to which the first Prime Minister of the PRC Zhou Enlai made an important contribution, was the attempt to break the bipolar scheme imposed by US imperialism.

Even the use of the term "superpower," which came into use in journalistic language, was deceptive, because it put the two countries on the same economic and military level, but they were not, in fact. The economic strength of the USSR – which had undoubtedly made great strides thanks to socialist planning in the 1930s and later – was nevertheless considerably less than that of the USA (and it should be remembered what a huge tribute of victims and economic destruction the USSR paid to defeat Nazi-Fascism, compared to the USA, which did not have war at home). The USSR was forced by the US offensive to the arms race, which allowed it a certain dissuasive power in the use of nuclear weapons, but not to reach parity with the US, which had the most powerful military-industrial complex in the world. Furthermore, the arms race to which the USSR was forced, diverted resources that could have been used in social spending to improve the standard of living and well-being of the people, thus weakening the consensus to the Soviet government and the Communist Party of the Soviet Union (CPSU). The USSR was not a "superpower," this label favored the ideological campaign to demonize it as an "empire of evil."

If we observe the historical experience of the defeat of Soviet socialism and European socialism, it can be seen that the terrain of confrontation of bipolarism imposed by the USA in the aftermath of the Second World War was favourable to the latter, which could pass after 1991 to the affirmation of unipolarism, of the USA as the only dominant centre in the world. Throughout the historical phase of the thirty years after 1991, the political and cultural forces of socialism, as well as of anti-colonial and anti-imperialist emancipation, proposed and fought for the end of US unipolarism and the transition to a multipolar world. This concept is not only opposed to unipolarism, but also to bipolarism, it rejects the "Cold War" battleground chosen by the imperialists. Holding the flag of the multipolar world, the world strategy of struggle for socialism learns the lessons of the historical experience of the twentieth century, understands that the world of the twenty-first century is articulated in different countries with different degrees of development of productive forces and relations of production with their respective political superstructures, the transition to more advanced socialist production relations cannot take place simultaneously, nor with a general final clash between the poles of socialism and imperialism, but through the combination of the consolidation and growth of socialist-oriented countries (and here the role of the PRC and socialism with Chinese characteristics is extremely important), with the escape from underdevelopment and dependence on imperialism of the countries of Asia, Africa and Latin America, with the class struggle between capital and labour in European capitalist countries, and a plurality of other intermediate social forms. The multipolar world would allow more favorable conditions for the transition to more advanced relations on the road to social emancipation and socialism.

The Belt and Road Initiative (BRI) is heading in the direction of a multipolar world, which builds fundamental infrastructures, creating the conditions for communication and mutual benefit for countries with different cultures, economic systems and political regimes, such as, for example, the growing commercial but also cultural relations between China and the EU, whose countries are for the most part affiliated to NATO, which is fully US-led.

The current policy of the US administration, which sees its unipolar domination increasingly staggering, is instead aiming at re-proposing the bipolarism scheme, which was successful during the "Cold War" period, and is trying to bring the PRC onto this ground. This is clearly shown by the increasingly frequent either-or (the heaviest is, as we have seen, that of Springer's CEO): European countries must choose, either with the USA or China. With bipolarism the US, fierce opponents of the BRI, tend to align European countries against the PRC under their command.

VIII. A difficult and complex world phase is opening

The forces of socialism and progress in the world are today called to the difficult task of opposing, also at the media level, the current US strategy, which aims at a bipolar US-China confrontation, presenting the latter as a "superpower." China has never said that it is or wants to become a "superpower." On the contrary, it has always said the opposite. And this is based on all the political thinking of the CPC, from Mao Zedong to Zhou Enlai, to Deng Xiaoping, to Xi Jinping. Underlying this is a well-established world view and strategic vision, which Xi's thought has further developed. It is the idea of a long and complex process of transition to socialism. China is today one of the main bastions for world peace, it is based on the idea of peaceful development. In the multipolar world one can play with a plurality of actors and contradictions. Socialist forces can move forward, as in fact has happened extraordinarily with the growth of China, Vietnam and Cuba. The bipolar world forces to clash wall against wall, forcing even the neutrals to take their place. It favors imperialism, with its enormous control over the media.

The new world situation determined by the COVID-19 pandemic and its political, cultural and social implications is still open to different solutions, to a possible progressive outlet for humanity. But the conservative and reactionary forces at world level, and in particular US imperialism, are decisively opposed to any possible community of shared destiny for all humanity. The current dominant class in the USA, born and raised in the culture of the American imperial mission and unchallenged domination over the whole world, does not accept the passage to a multipolar world, based on cooperation with mutual advantage between countries and blocs of countries with equal dignity. To the constructive and reasonable proposals of the PRC for world health cooperation, it responds with an escalation of real declarations of war, increasingly raising the level of the clash and trying to drag the PRC on the preferred terrain of clash of the USA. The bipolar confrontation allows the USA mobilizing the whole system of political-military alliances grown with the Cold War, first of all NATO, to yoke the European countries in the clash against China.

It opens a difficult and complex world phase, in which the forces of socialism, progress and social emancipation, which today have a fundamental point of reference in the PRC, have the historic task of strengthening international cooperation and solidarity and of countering with strategic political intelligence and tactical flexibility the forces of the imperialist reaction, working actively along the traced path of building a community of shared future for all humanity.

Different Systemic Approaches to the Pandemic in the World – the Question of Life and Death

[Czech Republic] Ming Liangsi

Edited by Tang Fangfang[1]

About the Author

Ming Liangsi is an expert on international and global relations; he focuses on PR China, the European Union, the USA and other major powers; the Belt and Road Initiative, etc.

Abstract

The article analyses the contemporary pandemic problems in their complex political, economic and social relations in global interactions in a historical trajectory from the past to the possible future development. It proceeds in five steps. First, it examines different systemic approaches to the COVID-19 pandemic in various parts of the world, including China's approach and the US approach of neoliberal capitalism. Second, it deals with the US-China trade frictions in the global interactions which are preconditions of the current pandemic and post-pandemic US-China disputes. Third, it analyses how the Belt and Road Initiative follows the conception of socialism developed

---

1   Tang Fangfang, assistant research fellow of the Academy of Marxism, Chinese Academy of Social Sciences.

by China's reform and opening up. The article explains that political, economic and social problems associated with the pandemic can be solved only if we understand how these problems are situated in historical regional and global interactions and how it can be improved and developed in the future.

The contemporary pandemic is a problem for all of humanity, as it affects many people and it can affect also many others. Even if humanity has already much historical experience with pandemics, it is still difficult to deal with it today. On the one hand, humanity has more scientific and organizational knowledge in the fight against a pandemic. On the other hand, last decades we live in a very complex and globally interconnected society, which allows for a faster spread of a pandemic. The faster humanity globalizes, the more often it runs into unexpected risks, as societies are not yet fully ready for this rapid development (Beck 2016).[1] Therefore, it is necessary to establish global interactions more thoroughly from the local level, through the national, regional and macro-regional levels to the global level. The interconnections of these levels would make possible better sustainable and cooperative interactions among societies. I will explain in this article that China with its global partners has already started developing this model of interactions.

Scientific research on the coronavirus pandemic and the COVID-19 disease is still underway. We have some knowledge about it, we can compare it with various respiratory diseases and other top causes of death,[2] and we know many

---

1   Ulrich Beck analysed global interactions as a world risk society (Beck 1999) which he later developed concerning unintended consequences of the development and also emancipatory tendencies of the problematic events.

2   World Health Organization (WHO), "Global Research on Coronavirus Disease (COVID-19)," April 30, 2020, see https://www.who.int/emergencies/diseases/novel-coronavirus-2019/global-research-on-novel-coronavirus-2019-ncov; WHO, "The Top 10 Causes of Death," May 24, 2018, see https://www.who.int/news-room/fact-sheets/detail/the-top-10-causes-of-death; WHO, "Up to 650 000 People Die of Respiratory Diseases Linked to Seasonal Flu Each Year," December 14, 2017, see https://www.who.int/news-room/detail/14-12-2017-up-to-650-000-people-die-of-respiratory-diseases-linked-to-seasonal-flu-each-year.

consequences caused by the pandemic. It almost stopped the economy and society in many parts of the world. Many governments, organizations and citizens have tried to fight the pandemic together. China, the World Health Organization, other UN agencies and many other countries and organizations have worked together even if some other countries with different approaches did not join the global efforts.

Various approaches to the pandemic are based on different political-economic systems, including "socialism with Chinese characteristics" and the Anglo-American approach of "neoliberal capitalism." It is necessary to understand that the pandemic disputes on public health between the US and China are a continuation of the US-China trade frictions by other means. In recent years, these two countries with their systems have come into clashes when the US President with his team began implementing global frictions. This is a reassessment of the current model of globalization, which the United States and the UK began to develop in the 1980s. In order to find a way out of this problem, now it is important to understand how China has contributed to the positive aspects of current globalization by its own model of global interactions mainly in the last two decades, and how this model can be further developed in the future. Closely related to this is an issue of how this China's model has recently developed by cooperation in various regions and macro-regions of the world, and how it can be further developed in the future. This means that it is relevant to analyse the current problems related to the pandemic not superficially in isolation and not only in the present in an ahistorical way. It is necessary to understand these issues in their complex economic and political relations in a historical trajectory from the past to the future.

Therefore, as for a methodology of this article, I focus on historical trajectory of the issue because only when we base theoretical and empirical analyses on a historical methodology, we can reach a deeper and sufficient understanding of the issue. There are several main streams of interpretation in China and Europe that follow a historical methodology. In China, first, there is a materialist historical methodology integral to the Marxist tradition; secondly, in the past of China, stretching back for more than two and a half thousand years, historical analyses have been considered an essential part of traditional schools of knowledge. Also in Europe, historical analyses have played a highly relevant role in empirical and theoretical works.

Particularly in this article, I proceed in five steps. In the first part, I examine different systemic approaches to the COVID-19 pandemic in various parts of the world. I distinguish three main approaches, and I also deal with a new technological approach. In the second part, I deal with the US-China trade frictions in the global interactions as preconditions of the current disputes in the pandemic and post-pandemic times which worsen the situation. In the third part, I show that China has various opportunities for cooperation in the world and that, therefore, it is not dominantly dependent on the United States. Specifically, I explain how China has gradually developed its own version of global interactions, i.e. the Belt and Road Initiative, which makes greater and fairer cooperation than the older Western version of globalization. It is the Belt and Road based on regional and macro-regional cooperation that can be taken into the future. In the fourth part, I show the sources of the Belt and Road Initiative, i.e. the contemporary Chinese conception of socialism developed by China's reform and opening up since 1978 which led to the global opening of China based on domestic reforms in China. Finally, in the fifth part of my article, I deal with one of fruitful specifications of the Belt and Road by explaining the cooperation with former socialist countries in Central and Eastern Europe, which now have developed social state, i.e. welfare state. Particularly, I would like to contribute to the overall understanding of the topic of the pandemic disputes among socialist and capitalist countries by showing how it can be perceived from the point of view of Central Europe.

The economic, political and social problems associated with a pandemic can only be overcome if we understand how these problems are situated in historical regional, macro-regional and global interactions and how these interactions can be developed positively in the future.

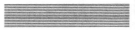

I. Different Systems, Different Approaches

Governments in different parts of the world have chosen different approaches to the pandemic. However, there are only a few basic approaches, and a range of options among them. I will explain three basic approaches, with the first and third contrasting with each other and the second approach standing between them.[1] The first approach was taken by PR China on the basis of its ability to pursue its socialist model which combines the market with strategic state planning and regulation and, then, some other countries followed the approach in the similar ways. The third approach is neoliberal capitalism represented mainly by the USA and the UK. Between them, there is the second approach which is characterized by the fact that at first some countries did not introduce the antivirus measures in time, for example Italy, and then it was too late to manage the situation even though the measures were strictly taken.

The first approach is to adopt restrictive measures, with the closure of infected areas, curfews, the wearing of masks, shutting down production, shops, etc. in order to protect public health. This approach has been introduced by China. Some European countries have followed suit, some partner countries in 17+1 Cooperation, for example, i.e. 17 countries of Central and Eastern Europe cooperating with China. Czechia and Slovakia, welfare states in Central Europe, got the information about the virus, and initially waited for the right time for antivirus measures not to come too quickly or too late. Czechia was one of the first countries in Europe to respond with strict measures. Other neighbouring European countries reacted similarly. As a result, the number of infected people and death toll are relatively small compared to Western European countries.

One of the reasons why most Central and Eastern European countries have

---

1   I analysed several approaches with a focus on a regrouping of global political and economic forces shortly in the Czech language in the *Literarni noviny* newspaper.

few infected people and deaths is probably also the fact that these countries built an extensive network of hospitals with free medical care during their socialist era and gradually modernized this network. The number of intensive care beds in the Czech Republic is larger than in Italy, for example, although Italy is six times larger than the Czech Republic concerning a population, and Italy is considered a developed Western country. Another probable reason for the relatively small number of infected people and deaths in Central Europe is that, in the socialist era, the whole population (children and adults) was systematically vaccinated against other diseases, such as tuberculosis. The vaccination complex could now be a suitable immune source of resistance in the Central European population. So far, however, this is only a hypothesis that needs to be verified.

Other countries in continental Europe subsequently responded with their government measures, similarly to the Czech Republic and Slovakia. What is remarkable is the comparison with Germany, which, as a relatively large country, is highly infected (around the 8th place in the world in May 2020),[1] but compared to other Western countries per capita it has (probably due to advanced organized health care, other welfare state measures and perhaps also the vaccination of the population of the former socialist East Germany) three to four times fewer deaths.[2]

As for the second group of countries with a different approach to the pandemic, the European countries with the most infected people in Europe, especially Italy and Spain, reacted late. Then, although they adopted strict measures as in China, these could no longer have the optimum effect even though their introduction in Italy was particularly severe. France, Russia and Brazil also did not initially estimate the situation, and are now among the most infected countries, despite the measures

---

1　"COVID-19 Coronavirus Pandemic," May 30, 2020, see https://www.worldometers.info/coronavirus/.
2　G. Gotev, "The Briefls Eastern Europe More Resilient to COVID-19?", *Euractiv*, April 2020, see https://www.euractiv.com/section/coronavirus/news/the-brief-is-eastern-europe-more-resilient-to-covid-19/.

taken. Similarly, they initially underestimated the virus in Turkey and Iran, where today, despite restrictions, there are most infected people in Muslim countries. But in Arab countries, they have better results. The situation seems to be similar in sub-Saharan Africa but the situation so far looks relatively favourable rather due to the small number of tests and the small record of the problem, with the risk of massive spread.

The third group of countries are those with a system of neoliberal capitalism, whose governments underestimate social problems and public health care the most. When the pandemic started, the USA and UK conservative governments initially adopted a relaxed laisser-faire approach. It did not resolve the situation there and, after announcing an initial estimate of 200,000 deaths in relation to a planned "herd immunity" strategy, under public pressure the British government was forced to reconsider its approach and tighten its rules, still leaving an estimated death toll of almost 40,000 (Boseley 2020) which became the reality in May 2020. This is the second highest death toll of all countries in the world, immediately after the US, where the situation in terms of infected people and dead toll is the worst globally (Worldometers 2020). Neoliberal capitalism has its fatal consequences. It is the deadliest regime in the world now.

The US neoliberal capitalist approach hit the poor and Afro-Americans the most. Racist policy brutality killed black people several times which caused demonstrations. Especially after George Floyd's death, protests erupted in Minneapolis, then escalated across the USA in dozens of cities and led to clashes with police[1]. The Pentagon ordered the army to prepare military police. In the UK, the black people are affected also much more. Coronavirus patients died at double

---

1 Editor, "Live Updates on George Floyd Protests: Pentagon Orders Army Units to Stand By," *New York Times,* May 30, 2020.

the rate of white in hospitals.[1] The poor are hit seriously as well.

There is another, technological measure which is linked to the first approach applied in China. The new technological measure has already proved successful in East Asia, particularly in PR China, Singapore, South Korea and other countries. In the fight against the pandemic, more and more politicians and citizens have begun to take this measure as a temporary solution. Some other countries implemented this measure on their own later. The Czech Republic, for example, introduced so called smart quarantine and other technological applications for tracing infected people with their contacts, etc. Tracing the contacts of infected people allows, among other things, the use of more adequate language, as we are talking about who became the mediator of the transmission of the virus to someone else. Otherwise, it is often said in abstract terms that "the virus is spreading" which is attributed to its greatly exaggerated abilities. Although the virus can slowly spread to a limited extent on its own, we give it the main dynamics of transmission by spreading it on ourselves and within ourselves by cars, planes, ships and other means globally beyond its capabilities.

The technological measure needs to be seen in the broader context of people being willing to take various measures in the struggle for survival and health, including widespread quarantine, wearing face masks, closing production, shops, offices, schools, etc. This is not only a struggle for survival but also a struggle for recognition as human beings who want to be respected as those who protect their loved ones and others around them. Nevertheless, it is sometimes recalled that a similar digital technology have often been seen in Europe and the USA as an invasion of privacy, in contrast to East Asian societies, where the penetration of digitalisation into people's lives is greater. At the same time, however, surprisingly the willingness of citizens of European countries and the USA to provide their data

---

1 A. Norfolk, "Black Coronavirus Patients Are Dying At Double The Rate Of WhiteIn Hospitals," *The Times*, April 24, 2020, see https://www.thetimes.co.uk/article/black-coronavirus-patients-are-dying-at-double-the-rate-of-white-in-hospitals-lddtfs6vz.

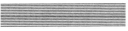

to entertainment social networks (Facebook, Twitter, etc.) is forgotten.

The use of new technologies is not an isolated phenomenon. It seems clear that we are entering the next stage of a new era, made possible by the pandemic. Otherwise, people's caution in taking technological measures would probably be much greater. Similar approaches are likely to be required in the events of future natural disasters related to climate change. The pandemic has just taken another step in this direction. Increasing human intervention in the wild – such as the deforestation of the Amazon rainforest and massive industrialized agriculture – is linked to the spread of various viruses to the human population and the emergence of epidemics. Human beings in the wild encounter species of viruses that previously remained separated from humans.[1] In addition, the melting of permafrost hides historical pathogens that are probably waiting for us in other epidemics or pandemics.

Gradual changes in the environment due to human intervention have intensified through the emergence and development of industrial society in modern times, it is a much longer-term problem in the thousands of years, which began with the establishment of human civilization,[2] especially the Western civilization. Long-term natural cycles (alternating ice and interglacial periods as well as smaller cycles) and irregular events on the planet also play a role here.

II. The USA-China Frictions in the Global Interactions

Individual countries and groups of countries did not take the explained

---

1   S. Shan, "Think Exotic Animals Are to Blame for the Coronavirus? Think Again," *The Nation*, February 18, 2020, see https://www.thenation.com/article/environment/coronavirus-habitat-loss; S. Shan,"Accelerating Habitat Loss Behind COVID-19. The Microbes, the Animals and Us," *Le monde diplomatique*, March 2020, see https://mondediplo.com/2020/03/05coronavirus; O.Susa, "Global Risks and Conflicts: the Social, Environmental, and Political Consequences," *Critical Sociology*, Vol. 45, No. 6, 2019, pp. 829-843.
2   Ming Liangsi, "Social And Environmental Conflicts Or Sustainable Development?", *Civitas*, 2019, Vol. 19, No. 2, pp. 281-295.

antivirus approaches in isolation but in global economic and political interactions, some of which were already developing in tensions before the pandemic. The pandemic only accelerated history. Like in cases of other similar historical events, a magnifying glass of the pandemic makes possible to see increased existing positives and negatives of regimes in various countries and in the world order. It is why neither the US-China trade frictions nor related global interactions have been expected to improve during the pandemic.

The fact that the USA system has not had the pandemic under control is a symbol of another stage of its declining economic and political power. The USA and some Western countries are strongly connected to the old model of globalization that they began to develop in the beginning of the 1980s. But four decades have passed since then, and the world has changed. The old model has already reached its limits several times. The last time, it was the 2008 financial and economic crisis.

Because the USA has been a declining power already before the pandemic, it tries to contain successful China mainly in economic and technological ways. The US politicians are using the pandemic as an excuse for greater decoupling with China. They also seek to discourage various countries from cooperating with China now. Some may actually bow. But most countries already see which political-economic system is better in last decades. They also see which system is capable of coping with the coronavirus crisis and which system is not. As I already mentioned, the United States is the worst country in the world when it comes to pandemic control.

China has a different historical record. China was able to participate in the current model of globalization last decades, develop itself and become the second biggest world economy in Nominal GDP, and maintain its autonomous economic and political system. The reform and opening up since 1978 took root and transformed China. Especially since the beginning of the new millennium, China has gradually become more active in the world, including a membership in WTO in 2001. It has been able to cope with the 2008 financial crises, also because national debt of China in relation to GDP is much lower than in the US and many other Western countries. In 2014, this was the first time in more than 140 years (since 1872) that the USA had lost its primacy as for China's share of world GDP (Purchasing Power Parity, PPP for short). Now China is back to the world stage as a major country and civilization. It will be an advantage in the post-pandemic times. In the contemporary era of profound world changes, China is much better prepared for the coming period of time.

China has cooperated closely with various agencies of the United Nations as well. It has also begun building its own contribution to realizing globalization in a more cooperative and developmental way. Due to the previous era and also due to the pandemic experience, some countries want to reshape globalization. They see that the first version of globalization, which was initiated by the USA and the UK decades ago, has delivered not only beneficial strong global economic interconnections but also triggered various problems and financial and economic crises around the world.

Developing countries in particular see that China has managed to develop its infrastructure and lift more than 800 million people out of poverty over the last 40 years. In addition, China has developed its high-tech economy and society. There is no doubt that the motivation for cooperation with China exists for developing and developed countries around the world. This is a good starting point for the post-pandemic era.

The coronavirus is sometimes simply said to be egalitarian. But the fact is that although every person can be infected, poorer people in particular have worse living and working conditions, in which they are more likely to be infected than higher income groups.[1] The situation is problematic in developing countries, where many people lack adequate supplies of drinking water and soap, for example, especially

---

1   United Nations Global Compact, "Poverty," April 30, 2020, see https://www.unglobalcompact. org/what-is-gc/our-work/social/poverty; World Food Program, "2020: Global Report on Food Crises," April 20, 2020, see https://www.wfp.org/publications/2020-global-report-food-crises.

in the favelas and slums. Oxfam estimates that another half billion people may be put into poverty due to the coronavirus pandemic, unless measures are taken to help developing countries now (Oxfam 2020). The coronavirus therefore reproduces current inequalities and sometimes exacerbates them, especially when it arouses intolerance and racism instead of solidarity.

China proved that it cooperated with its foreign partners in full solidarity in the pandemic crisis. It delivered coronavirus medical aid to many countries in Asia, Africa, the Americas, and Europe. In Africa, China helped a modernization of the African Centre for Disease Control and Prevention, and sent protective equipment to many countries there, to Ethiopia, Ghana, and South Africa, for example.[1] In Europe, China sent masks, respirators and other medical material and equipment to Italy and other hit countries. European Commission President, Ursula von der Leyen, said "we were grateful for China's support the EU against COVID-19, and that we needed each other's help in times of need."[2]

The short-term consequences of the pandemic mean that economic activity has slowed more than in the 2008 financial crisis, but it may not be drastic in the long run. The positive side is the difference between today's pandemic situation and the situation of the 2008 financial and economic crisis. On the one side, this time economic activities almost stopped in many countries in a short run as a consequence of the pandemic which was a bigger impact than in the 2008 global financial crisis. However, there is no economic reason of the economic slowdown now. It is a non-economic viral cause. Therefore, as soon as the viral cause disappears step by step, hypothetically taken, global economy can rebound almost fully to its original state in the long-term. It already started revitalizing in many

1 S. Ebrahim, "China is Lending Africa a Hand during the COVID-19 Pandemic," *IOL*, May 7, 2020, see https://www.iol.co.za/news/opinion/watch-china-is-lending-africa-a-hand-during-the-covid-19-pandemic-47654517.
2 J. Valero, "EU Allocates Chinese Aid to Italy to Fight Against the Pandemic," *Euractiv*, March 19, 2020, see https://www.euractiv.com/section/coronavirus/news/eu-allocates-chinese-aid-to-italy-to-fight-against-the-pandemic/1444769/.

countries.

Nevertheless, things never return totally to their original state. A drop of GDP is expected in many countries in 2020, and next year is uncertain. An important factor in a pandemic is the fact that it spreads over the planet gradually, so that the negative economic impacts are phased and partially mitigated. While the pandemic wave is already coming to an end in China, Europe could soon be at its peak. After the China's economy slowed in the first quarter, it is now beginning to improve again. Next year it can regain its strength. But this will depend not only on Chinese companies, institutions and consumers, but also on how the global economy will develop, mainly in Europe and the US. In any event, China may be at a global advantage due to the time lag of the pandemic wave, because it is likely to resume its economic activities earlier than Western countries.

Temporarily, so-called de-globalization tendencies in production and trade may prevail, which may exacerbate the existing structural economic and financial problems of the global system, including the US-China trade frictions. However, it will still be a highly globalized future society when we compare it to how globalized it was decades ago. It will be rather a global reorganization than true de-globalization. Indeed, in history, globalization has always been dialectically contradictory within the waves of global integration, subsequent partial disintegration, and subsequent even larger global integration.

Because the USA has the worst consequences of the pandemic in the world, the seriousness of the situation is not underestimated by former US Secretary of State and National Security Adviser Henry Kissinger. In his article, "The Coronavirus Pandemic Will Forever Alter the World Order,"[1] he stresses the need to start preparing for a new different era. Even if he has in mind different needs

---

1   H.Kissinger, "The Coronavirus Pandemic Will Forever Alter the World Order," *Wall Street Journal*, April 3, 2020, see https://www.wsj.com/articles/the-coronavirus-pandemic-will-forever-alter-the-world-order-11585953005?fbclid=IwAR0A_06PmvRcRQV2umVY4TNcpY8AYctG3pOSpjGh2ww2Jk 1M47KoUAh8ZIs.

and interests, we can take this change positively as space for a better regrouping of global cooperation. China can build more on its own version of globalization, i.e. on the global Belt and Road Initiative (BRI), and intensify its cooperation with developed and developing countries in Eurasia, as well as with developing countries in Africa and Latin America, where cooperation and assistance are particularly needed.

III. The Belt and Road Initiative

The first version of globalisation, which the USA and the UK started to pursue in the 1980s and which is still working to some degree, delivered not only much more forceful global interconnection in various aspects, but also triggered problems and crises around the world. This took place in cycles of integration and disintegration waves, albeit against the backdrop of long-running global integration trends.

China is a developing country, or more precisely the biggest developing country, which contributes to global exchanges.[1] Yet China also offers something innovative: Globalisation 2.0. It is the China's Belt and Road Initiative which has brought, above all, a new stage of global interactions in the era of significant world changes.

The BRI, built along the ancient Silk Road and beyond, has made a relevant contribution as, historically, it stems from the unique long-term development of China's civilization, from the establishment of the PR China 70 years ago, and from China's reform and opening up in recent decades. The BRI has contributed significantly to the development and multipolarity of the world by efforts to

---

1   It is important to understand interconnections between China's internal development and global development. I plan to enlarge my analysis of this issue, which I touch in this and next sessions of this article, in my separated article focusing on the development from China's reform to the world's reform.

cooperate on the basis of mutual recognition of participating partners. Since it was announced by President Xi Jinping in 2013, the BRI has been developed as a model in Eurasia and Eastern Africa, it has also encompassed Latin America, it is a global project. It is already indicated in the concept of "a community of shared future for mankind."

It fits well the global tendencies of new alternatives. While we have recently witnessed faltering unilateralism, we can see China and other countries introducing a multipolar perspective. This is not limited to the BRICS countries but also includes Mexico, Indonesia, Turkey, for example, and also macro-regional initiatives, such as the European Union, the Eurasian Union, the Shanghai Cooperation Organization, etc. In fact, already the BRI's official names define a plurality of paths: the, Silk Road Economic Belt and the 21st Century Maritime Silk Road, with their various economic corridors and many projects, including infrastructure network and production capacity with various aspects. The Polar Silk Road may also be established in the Arctic at some point in the future.

The BRI introduces connectivity and makes investments in many countries, facilitating development in areas such as the economy, research and innovation, culture, and people-to-people communication, etc.

Over time, the BRI has become a publicly well-known programme on a global scale. In order to understand its essence and its potential for future development, we need to analyse it in relation to the resources that made it materially and conceptually possible. When researchers try to explain the specific motivation driving the establishment of the BRI at a specific moment in time, they see chronological coincidences with the consequences of the economic and financial crisis playing out almost globally since 2007 and 2008, particularly the crisis in the USA and other Western countries, which dragged the economies of many other countries down with them. Since the crisis erupted, Western countries' demand for Chinese goods has experienced a downtrend. As the Chinese economy was export-oriented, the Chinese government was keen to help Chinese companies at the time of crisis, and reverse the trend. Promoting and financially supporting public infrastructure and other projects in China as a counterbalance to the consequences of the global economic crisis, the Chinese government also started being active in the international and transnational spheres after several years of uncertainty on Western markets. The announcement of the Belt and Road Initiative in 2013 was a creative effort to reinvent the historical Silk Road in a new form appropriate for the 21st century. In the mass media environment of our era, positive and nostalgic connotations of the Silk Road, replete with camel caravans transporting the exotic goods on demand in Central Asia and Europe for almost two thousand years, captured the imagination and encapsulated the idea of the project of win-win cooperation.

The Belt and Road Initiative in general was already described well,[1] and it needs no big introduction. It is relevant to mention that, following China's economic opening up, China has signed more than BRI 100 agreements on cooperation with various countries and international organisations. Under the BRI, merchandise trade between the countries involved had exceeded $5 trillion by June 2018. In the first five years of the Initiative, China made a direct investment of more than $70 billion. As for engineering projects, the value of contracts signed is over $500 billion. The BRI has generated $2.01 billion in tax revenues and created 244,000 jobs.[2] The BRI's well-trodden economic development corridors connect Eurasia, and include the high-profile project of a railway connecting Budapest (Hungary) and Belgrade (Serbia) and later hopefully also the Piraeus Port in Athens, along with projects around the China-Pakistan Economic Corridor, to mention just a couple.

The people in these countries are aware of the results achieved by Chinese

---

1   Wang Y., *The Belt and Road Initiative. What Will China Offer the World in Its Rise,* Beijing: New World Press, 2016; Wang M., "Civilizations and its Conceptualizations in Ethnology, Social Anthropology, and Sociology," *Journal of China in Comparative Perspective,* Vol.3, No.1, 2017, pp.44-47.
2   Lu Y., "China's merchandise trade with Belt and Road countries tops $5 trillion in 5 years," *People's Daily,* August 31, 2018, see http://en.people.cn/n3/2018/0831/c90000-9496013.html.

developments to date. Not only has China become the world's largest economy by GDP PPP, but has also significantly increased the standard of living enjoyed by its population. In 1976, more than 82% of China's population lived in the countryside, most of them in poverty. Over the 40 years of China's reform and opening up, hundreds of millions people have been lifted from poverty. It is an unprecedented achievement in the history of mankind. Moreover, almost 400 million people on the east coast of China have a standard of living on a par with the average in the European Union. Developing countries are inspired by the Chinese model in the light of such statistics when they consider joining the Belt and Road Initiative. On top of that, many developed countries have come round to viewing China as an important partner for cooperation in recent decades.

Of course, any model is not ideal and includes limits which need to be overcome. It is important to stress that people support the BRI and are inspired by the Chinese model, in that they highlight how these initiatives contribute to positive developments. Set against the backdrop of the world's current problems, this is something that they identify as a positive component of multilateralism that deserves to be supported and furthered.

Now let's look at the necessary conditions giving rise to the BRI in the decades preceding its establishment, i.e. in China's era of reform and opening up starting in 1978. It shows how the Chinese internal model of "socialism with Chinese characteristics" is a basis of the Chinese model of globalization represented by BRI.

IV. China's reform and opening up

The Belt and Road Initiative follows China's reform and opening up. Thus, this initiative adopted by China was a logical consequence consistent with Chinese developments. This transformation and opening up, in tandem with previous historical developments, were relevant conditions of BRI. This is a sign that it is well deeply rooted in a chronological context. President Xi Jinping also mentioned elements of BRI in Chinese medium- and long-term history.[1] To articulate this approach generally, any truly unalienated innovation in society has to follow historically shaped needs, interests, values, and possibilities.

The fact that the BRI is based on international projects must be considered in close relation to the previous forty years of China's reform and opening up, starting in 1978. In that time, Deng Xiaoping had sought to develop a specific version of Chinese development. He knew that it would not be practical to copy another country's system because every country and, especially, every civilization is different.[2] Furthermore, he saw the Western system's long history of association with colonialism. Particularly in the 19th century and the first half of the 20th century, Western countries had expanded their colonies considerably by military force. The Western "democracies" then collapsed in fratricidal fighting in the First World War before hauling the world into the Second World War. The Western countries were then forced to relinquish their colonial territories, but did so reluctantly and, in the post-colonial period, made constant attempts to dominate the territories of their former colonies, and sometimes also deployed the military in doing so.

Deng Xiaoping was not willing to introduce this model in China. However, he did want to learn from developments in various parts of the world and use them as a source of inspiration.[3] From 1978, Deng Xiaoping started pursuing an approach that would be consistent with the new era of Chinese history: economic reform and opening up China to the world. The relationship between internal and external models is important here. While many developing countries were forced to accept the Western model in order to be allowed to cooperate with it globally, China was able to integrate itself into the global economy but, at the same time, to keep and

---

1   Xi Jinping, *The Governance of China II*, Beijing: Foreign Languages Press, 2017, pp. 543-566.
2   Deng Xiaoping, *Selected Works of Deng Xiaoping (1965-1982)*, ICP Intercultural Press, 2015.
3   E. F. Vogel, *The Four Little Dragons: The Spread of Industrialization in East Asia*, Harvard University Press, 1992; Yang B., *Deng: A Political Biography*, Armonk and London: M. E. Sharpe, 1998; P. Nolan, *China and the West: Crossroads of Civilization*, London and New York: Routledge, 2018, p.IX.

develop its own domestically more appropriate model. China's transformation and opening up as of 1978 laid the foundations for foreign efforts under the Belt and Road Initiative. 1978 was a very important year, and not just for China. Though each partner maintained its own system, there were certain system overlaps and new common areas. These interactions also changed the USA and European economies.[1] From the end of the 1990s, the Chinese government motivated Chinese companies to invest abroad with a "Go out policy." "Go global" gradually became the motto for Chinese interactions.

Martin Jacques considers 1978 one of the most relevant years in the 20th century.[2] I think it is the most important year of the 20th century. China came up with a concept that interlinks Western and Chinese elements to mould them into a specific new approach in practice. The Chinese concept took root and transformed China into the world's second largest economy (by nominal GDP). China's GDP was USD 150 billion in 1978, and is USD 14.2 trillion (nominal) in 2019, or approximately USD 27 trillion by PPP. Using GDP (PPP) as a basis, China became the world's largest economy at the turn of 2014. China's economy accounts for 19% of world output now. After two centuries, China is back on the world stage as a major country and civilization.

Crucially, this development triggered an unprecedented increase in the standard of living for more than a billion people in China and many other people across the world via the BRI. These are not just abstract statistics glossing over the plight of the people, particularly the poor. As I have indicated, in the past 40 years China has elevated 800 million people from poverty, and it has plans for remaining people to be lifted out of poverty by 2020 or 2021 and for solving other social

---

1 H.Schmidt and F. Sieren, *Nachbar China*, Berlin: Econ Verlag, 2006; Yang B., *Deng: A Political Biography*, Armonk and London: M. E. Sharpe, 1998.
2 M. Jacques, "Cambridge scholar lauds reform and opening up while underscoring West's ignorance of nation," *Global Times*, October 28, 2018, see http://www.globaltimes.cn/content/1124826.shtml.

issues.[1] This has meant a big improvement in social rights. If we take into account that China has 1.42 billion people (as of 2019 according to UN data), i.e. 18.4% of the world population, this social development is an enormous achievement in the history of human civilization. At the same time, the Chinese government knows that many people are still faced with more meagre standards of living, and it plans to improve the situation in the years to come. As China, thanks to its model of transformation and opening up to the world, has become a major global economy exercising a significant influence on the standard of living in China and, via the BRI, abroad, 1978 can be described as at least the most important year in the 20th century, and perhaps over a larger timescale.

There are several main reasons underpinning the successful transformation of China's economic system.[2] The core logic behind the Chinese reform and opening up of last 40 years was that international trade was not taking place between two countries employing the same system. The Western countries, on the one hand, and China, on the other, had different political and economic models. As David Daokui Li stresses, the fact that the Chinese government manages in an active way the economy has been considered a relevant factor for a rapid economic development.[3]

The socialist China had two salient features. First, as it was making significant investments in companies thanks to the rules of banks, it was reporting the large capital returns of a country. Unlike many Western-oriented countries where profit was accumulated and then often inefficiently spent, China also ploughed profits into social development. There are social projects designed to improve the situation,

1 Wang W., *Social Change in Contemporary China and the Theory of Social Contradictions*, Reading, UK: Paths International and China Social Sciences Press, 2015; Wang W., *Social Interests and Conflict: A Socialist Analysis of Contemporary China*, Reading, UK: Paths International and China Social Sciences Press, 2015.
2 Wei X., *Rethinking China's Economic Transformation*, New York: Global Scholarly Publications, 2010.
3 Li D., et al., *Economic Lessons Learned from China's Forty Years of Reform and Opening Up*, Beijing: Tsinghua University, 2018.

including in parts of China beyond the well-developed East Coast, and to foster a more egalitarian approach in the future.

Secondly, the Chinese economy's transformation was successful because of "big-country effect." Scope of economy is a determining factor. China is not just one of the successful small Asian tigers but it is characterized by an application of a more influential model: the Flying Dragon Model. This model changed a small, cheap production and trading partner into a major force, via learning through the history. A complex process of practical learning through opening up is more important here than individual aspects of reform, i.e. more than comparative advantage in relation to the West and dependence on foreign capital and technologies.[1] The Chinese meritocratic recognition of education and work plays a role here.

It was on the strength of this successful transformation of the Chinese economy that makes possible to refer to 1978 as the second revolution in China. As this is a revolution that did not occur immediately, but instead delivered significant changes over the course of several decades within a revolutionary reform.[2] The Belt and Road Initiative is one of important consequences of that development.

V. The Belt and Road and former socialist countries in Central and Eastern Europe

The Silk Road made an enormous contribution to global history through mutual inspiring interactions between the East and West. Without the Silk Road, other parts of Asia, Europe and Africa in particular would probably be different now because innovations travelled mainly from East (China, India, Persia, etc.) to

---

1 Li D., et al., *Economic Lessons Learned from China's Forty Years of Reform and Opening Up*, Beijing: Tsinghua University, 2018.
2 J. P. Arnason and M. Hrubec (eds.), *Social Transformations and Revolutions*, Edinburgh: Edinburgh University Press, 2016.

West.[1] The Belt and Road Initiative was proposed with the aim of building on the heritage of the Silk Road in a modern way. It is an ambitious programme aimed at intensifying connections, communication and cooperation among countries and regions in Euroasia[2] and also in Africa and Latin America. It respects the five principles of coexistence and mutual cooperation: respect for sovereignty, non-aggression, non-interference in internal affairs, equality and mutual benefit, and peaceful coexistence.

The announcement of the BRI followed on from a broader framework of efforts of President Xi Jinping who proposed concept of the Chinese Dream.[3] This concept is linked to the "great rejuvenation" of China, with chronological aims of a "moderately well-off society" by 2021 (the 100th anniversary of the foundation of CPC) and a developed society by 2049 (the 100th anniversary of the foundation of PR China), with a milestone in-between in 2035. This new epoch in the transformation of China, including the Belt and Road Initiative, is sometimes called the third revolution. Therefore, if we take 1911 as year zero for modern China, 1949 as the first revolution, and 1978 as the second revolution, we might view 2013 as the beginning of the third revolution because of the foundation of the Belt and Road Initiative and the related formulation of the Chinese Dream. We can see that these revolutions and revolutionary transformations have domestic and also some global consequences and their interconnections.

On the domestic issue, various problems are fought with more adequate regulation under new leadership in the current turbulent global era, with stronger leadership also present in other major countries. There is also support for domestic consumption in order to make the Chinese economy less dependent on Chinese

---

1 P. Frankopan, *The Silk Roads: A New History of the World*, New York: Vintage, 2017.
2 A. Lukin, "Sino-Russian Cooperation as the Basis for Greater Eurasia," *Human Affairs*, Vol. 30, No. 2, 2020, pp.174-188. I. Denisov, I.Safranchuk and D.Bochkov, "China-India Relations in Eurasia: Historical Legacy and Changing Global Context," *Human Affairs*, Vol. 30, No. 2, 2020, pp.224-238.
3 Xi Jinping, *The Governance of China*, Beijing: Foreign Languages Press, 2014, pp. 37-75.

exports, especially on the West, and particularly the USA. As for the global issue, Xi
Jinping has reformulated a foreign policy into a major cooperative project.[1] Along
the Belt and Road Initiative, the establishment of the Asia Infrastructure Bank as
a development bank for the financing of infrastructure in Asia and beyond was
announced in 2013. Since then, it has supplemented the activities of the World Bank
(WB) and the International Monetary Fund (IMF). Other projects followed.

The BRI stresses transnational and global production, trade, and other
cooperation, as well as domestic development, both linked to global interactions
with various macro-regions around the world and also focused on the mutual
interconnectedness of Chinese provinces in order to improve, in particular, the less-
developed Western provinces.

Since the BRI forges links among various places around the world, it focuses
primarily (1) on the overall territory of the Initiative, and (2) on particular macro-
regions and regions of the project.[2] While the 16+1 Cooperation, i.e. a cooperation
of 16 former socialist countries of Central and Eastern Europe with China, can be
understood in its narrower sense to pursue its own agenda since it was established
in 2012, it plays an important role in part of the BRI as well, which is supported by
the fact that Greece with its strategic Piraeus Port in Athens joined the Cooperation
and transformed it into the 17+1 Cooperation in 2019. The 16+1 Cooperation was
created originally to develop strategic dialogue and cooperation between PR China
and 16 ex-socialist Central and Eastern European Countries (CEECs). At the same
time, it has been defined in such a way that it is considered to be one of the BRI
parts focusing on a specific macro-region of the BRI. Both activities include various
types of projects in the fields of investment, energy, transport, trade, research,

---

1   Wu Z., "Functional Logic of the Belt and Road Initiative: Based on a New Interpretation of
Geoeconomics," *SASS Studies*, 2018, 12, pp.28-68.
2   Here I follow my comparative analyses of the Belt and Road Initiative in relation to the 16+1
Cooperation.

education, culture, environment, etc.[1] So far in the 17+1 Cooperation like in the BRI, China has stressed the importance of connectivity, infrastructure, etc. The 17+1 Cooperation holds annual summits of political leaders to set out step by step the cooperation, and a series of academic and other conferences. These activities have helped increasing contacts and collaboration and overcoming past isolation.

The BRI has a strong global aim in the UN global plan for the 2030 Agenda. The 17 Central and Eastern European countries aim to contribute to the 2030 Agenda as well. From this perspective, the 17+1 Cooperation can be viewed both as part of the 17 countries' contribution to the BRI and also as part of their own broader, global agenda. The BRI and the 17+1 Cooperation are ambitious projects. Of course, ambitious projects by definition also include various risks that have to be addressed. New challenges have been linked to the development and application of artificial intelligence, the 5G network, the internet of things, security and cyber-security, new social media, domestic and cross-border e-commerce, for example. Much will depend on how it will be used in order to satisfy the needs, interests and values of people in various local areas, countries, regions, macro-regions, and human civilization as a whole, and also in relation to the environment.

The 17+1 Cooperation and the BRI both attempt to bring more strategic dialogue, connectivity and cooperation to the territorial parts of these projects. Both projects are pursuing the ambition of bringing people and their activities together. While the 17+1 Cooperation focuses on the macro-region of Central Europe, the Baltic states, and the Balkans, and this macro-region's relations with China, the BRI Initiative focuses on the much larger territorial space of Asia, Europe, Africa, and Latin America. In both cases, China and its partners are developing long-term

---

1   Huang P. and Liu Z. (eds), *China-CEEC Cooperation and the "Belt and Road Initiative,"* Beijing: China Social Sciences Press, 2016; Huang P. and Liu Z. (eds), *How the 16+1 Cooperation Promotes the Belt and Road Initiative*, Beijing: China Social Sciences Press, 2017.

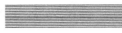

thinking and activities with international and transnational dimensions.[1]

VI. Conclusion: Against Racism and Intolerance

Tendayi Achiume, the UN Special Rapporteur on contemporary forms of racism, racial discrimination, xenophobia and related intolerance, has criticized the irresponsible and discriminatory state rhetoric of some Western politicians, mainly the US politicians, who have commented on the coronavirus pandemic in relation to some countries, particularly to China.[2] In agreement, Tedros Adhanom Ghebreyesus, Head of the World Health Organization, has demanded that the pandemic should not be politicized in this way.[3] As the USA is a failed state in dealing with the pandemic, its government should admit that it is necessary to go a different way.

We can learn from the political and economic problems of the coronavirus pandemic, and emancipate ourselves from these problems. Together as humanity, we can manage the pandemic this time and also next times: its health risks, social and economic problems, and political and environmental challenges. In order to do so, we have to understand the issue in the historical framework of global interactions from the past to the future.

China's global Belt and Road Initiative, as a new model of interactions, from local to global, can help overcoming the contemporary US-China trade frictions and developing fully a new kind of global interactions based on better connectivity, cooperation and justice. The Belt and Road Initiative involves historical

---

1   Ming Liangsi, "Approaches of the EU Towards the 16+1 Cooperation: Three Cases in the Framework of the Belt and Road Initiative," in Huang Ping, Liu Zuokui (eds), *16+1 Cooperation and the Belt and Road Initiative: Europe's Responses*, Beijing: China Social Sciences Press, 2018, pp. 97-108.

2   P. Kenny, "UN expert hits out at COVID-19 xenophobia," *AA*, March 3, 2020, see https://www.aa.com.tr/en/latest-on-coronavirus-outbreak/un-expert-hits-out-at-COVID-19-xenophobia/1776554.

3   UN News, "No need to politicize COVID-19," April 8, 2020, see https://news.un.org/en/story/2020/04/1061392.

preconditions: not only the impetus of the 2008 financial and economic crisis, but also deeper historical sources. It follows also on from the more than 40 years of China's reform and opening up since 1978 which made socialism with Chinese characteristics possible and has opened China to the world.

Following on from these historical developments in China and the old Silk Road, the Belt and Road Initiative has made a specific contribution to the multilateral global community when we consider various local, national, regional and macro-regional needs, interests and values in various parts of the world in their specific modalities and civilizations, and also in relation to human civilization in general. The 17+1 Cooperation, as a platform of fruitful interactions between Central and Eastern European countries and China, is an example of the cooperative specification of the Belt and Road Initiative in one of the world macro-regions. It is the opposite of the US-China tensions even if also some countries of the 17+1 Cooperation will have to face various challenges interlinked to these tensions which will try to limit development of the 17+1.

Of course, there have also clearly been challenges that need to be overcome by all the participants, as in any endeavour, in Central Europe and also more generally in the 17+1 Cooperation and within the BRI. Members of the 17+1 will continue their attempts to find a consensus also with partners in Western countries of the European Union and beyond. The BRI members will communicate with their partners also together with China. A new arrangement for relations with the USA and the development of relations with BRICS countries and other major and smaller countries will be needed in relation to the BRI in order to make a significant contribution to the global development in the post-pandemic times.

The Success of the Socialist System in the Face of the Emergency Caused by the Spread of COVID-19

[Italy] Francesco Marigiò

Edited by Li Kaixuan[1]

About the Author

Francesco Maringiò is a member of the Central Committee of the Italian Communist Party, and president of Italy Association for the Promotion of New Silk Road. He also serves as a foreign commentator for Xinhua News Agency, China Radio International and China Central Television. He is one of the founding members of Political-Cultural Association Marx XXI (Associazione Politico-Culturale Marx XXI), and organized the publishing of *Interviews with Chinese Marxists (Interviste ai marxisti cinesi,* 2017), a collection of the interviews with scholars from the Academy of Marxism at the Chinese Academy of Social Sciences. He is also one of the chief editors of the Italian version of *China in the New Era (La Cina nella nuova era,* 2019).

---

1 Li Kaixuan, associate research fellow of the Academy of Marxism, Chinese Academy of Social Sciences.

Abstract

The emergency management systems for responding to the COVID-19 pandemic can be divided into two models: the model of socialist China which places human life at the center of its initiative and the model of capitalist countries which is oriented towards the defense of private profit in spite of the health and life of their citizens. The success of China's model attracts worldwide attention, and also accounts for why the US, which has expressed a loss of interest in playing a leading role in global affairs in recent years, plays a main part in the new round of activities intended to counter China. In Italy, a transversal "anti-Chinese party" is soon organized when the public opinions in Italy express the wish to enter into an alliance with China beyond the Atlantic Alliance. At present, the destructiveness of anti-China topics deserves close attention of main think tanks and political heavyweights in all countries.

The world that will emerge when the virus will be eradicated will be different from the one that previously existed. Although of course it will not lead to a total overturning of the international balance of power, the leading capitalist countries behave as if this eventuality would be imminent. What the Chinese government's management of COVID-19 teaches us and what impact it can have on world public opinion.

The field of capitalist and imperialist countries is shifting humanity's struggle against the spread of COVID-19 into a global dispute against China and socialism.

In a first moment, when the reported and recognised cases of the virus were all inside China, we witnessed an unprecedented speculation. In fact, if we rewind the tape of the news that the mainstream media system gave us during the crucial weeks of the virus' spread in Wuhan, we would be reminded of the articles published by the *New York Times*, *Reuters* and other big news agencies (and promptly reported by the European media) that first complained to the Beijing authorities about the alleged delays and then claimed that the containment and quarantine measures were violating people's individual freedoms.

No empathy in the face of the health emergency, no human solidarity constraints, on the contrary: what was presented to the public at large was the spread of the stigma of the anointing for an entire population. All the above, it is important not to forget, acted as an explosive mixture for the spread of offensive clichés and racist stereotypes. At the expense of an entire population affected by the virus and its community of people living abroad who have been subject to aggression and discrimination. "Chinese virus" was written in hashtags on social networks, precisely to mark the blame towards China which has become in the mainstream story "the real sick man of Asia"[1] (the ignoble definition is from the *Wall Street Journal*): exactly the same expression used in a derogatory way at the end of the 19th and beginning of the 20th century to refer to China, divided and subjugated by colonial powers.

In a second moment, when there were cases of COVID-19 outside of China, Western media and policymakers shifted the attention to the alleged responsibility of China and the Chinese Communist Party in the spread of the virus, despite the fact that Beijing had already made available the knowledge and information acquired on this new pneumonia and offered its help to several countries of the European Union (EU) (starting from Italy).

The reason for this troubled relationship of the media as well as the governments of capitalist and imperialist countries with China consists in the success that the socialist country has achieved in the fight against the COVID-19 pandemic: on 31 December 2019 China reported to the international community the presence of some pneumonia outbreaks of unknown aetiology which, a few days later, was identified as Sars-CoV-2 Coronavirus. Since 23 January 2020 Wuhan has been quarantined, on 30 January the World Health Organization (WHO) declared

---

1   "China Is the Real Sick Man of Asia," *Wall Street Journal*, March 2, 2020, see https://www.wsj.com/articles/china-is-the-real-sick-man-of-asia-11580773677.

the Coronavirus as a "public health emergency of international concern" and then "pandemic" from 11 March 2020. On March 18 there were zero cases of new infection in Wuhan and, after 76 days of lockdown, the city reopened.

I. The universality of the Chinese health system during emergencies

A country's systemic response to a sanitary emergency can be determined by the contribution of three drivers: the existence of health infrastructure, scientific knowledge and the state of health of the population. As these components increase, there is a greater capacity for systemic response to the emergency. To sum up, we can say that the key to better tackle the challenges caused by a health crisis lies in the ability of public institutions to intervene structurally on the health, education and Research and Development (R&D) levels, given that the successes recorded today are the result of a transfer of knowledge from entire previous generations that can be used today.[1]

Another key factor is the overall level of economic equality. Indeed, several studies have shown that only by reducing inequalities can the institutional capacity to use public resources in the collective interest be increased. Conversely, the growth of inequalities leads to a weakening of state institutions and the distortion of public resources in favour of particular private interests. China's rise over the last 40 years has indeed brought about inequalities and polarisation of wealth, but as this story suggests, the difference with Western countries is visible precisely in the independence of political decision-makers from the profit maximisation demands of the private sector, which has indeed been co-opted and driven by political power in

---

1   This vision of technological progress is different between socialist and capitalist countries. In the latter, emphasis is placed on the action taken by individuals, which press and media turn into myths, thus obscuring the collective, often public, role actually played in technological progress.

the fight against COVID-19.[1] We shall return to this point later.

All these factors are very interesting and we can also use them as a paradigm for a deeper understanding of contemporary China. In fact, although in China there is not yet a public health system based on the principles of universality, equality and equity (as in the Italian model) and a level of welfare state that is still lower than that provided in Western European countries (although it is now under attack by the capitalist ruling classes),[2] the Chinese government's systemic response has been very high and efficient. The state response has enabled China to strengthen its health infrastructure, raise the level of health and education of the population and increase scientific knowledge, thus laying the foundations for promptly limiting the spread of the virus and reducing its mortality rate.

The progressive advancement of the private-sector role (also in the healthcare sector) over the last 40 years has not undermined the state's ability to increase research and healthcare spending,[3] also to balance the inequalities in medical access that have been recorded over time and which has led to a relative worsening of the poorest sections of the population.

When the outbreak of the virus broke out, we received news from the United

---

1   "Alibaba Cloud has offered AI computing capabilities to public research institutions for free to support virus gene sequencing, new drug R&D and protein screenings. Baidu has opened up LinearFold, its RNA prediction algorithm, to genetic testing agencies, epidemic prevention centres and research institutes around the world. Neusoft Medical donated high-end CT scanners, AI medical imaging, cloud platform and remote advanced post-processing software to hospitals in Wuhan. Infervision launched a 'Coronavirus AI solution,' an AI software for front-line clinicians to detect and monitor the disease on CT scans." Taken from: David Aikman and Alan Chan, "Five ways Chinese companies are responding to coronavirus," in World Economic Forum, https://www.weforum.org/agenda/2020/02/coronavirus-chinese-companies-response/.

2   See: J.P.Morgan, "The Euro area adjustment: about halfway there," May 28, 2013, which calls for the suppression of anti-fascist Constitutions contaminated by socialist ideas and the reduction of the welfare state. The document has raised fierce controversy and can no longer be viewed on the Bank's website. However, it can be found on the web, among others, at this address: https://www.europe-solidarity.eu/documents/ES1_euro-area-adjustment.pdf.

3   Over the last 40 years China has seen an increase in the healthcare expenditure-to-GDP ratio from 3 to 6.43% in 2018 compared to 1978 (although the population has increased by 45%).

States that testing for the coronavirus could cost more than $3,000 per citizen. We know, however, that the virus-infected population in China has been able to rely on a national welfare system that has borne all the costs: the central government, together with local governments, has covered the expenses of the treatment of all affected citizens, for an investment of over 2 billion euros. While outside the epicentre, efforts have been made to reduce infection to a minimum, more resources have been put in place to fight the virus in the epicentre: new beds and hospitals have been set up (12,000 patients can be placed in buildings temporarily converted into hospitals and 5,000 patients can be admitted to the two new hospitals built in about ten days). 300 teams of doctors were mobilised throughout the country, involving more than 40,000 staff, sent to the front line in the epicentre and the government gave them financial subsidies (RMB 6,000) and asked for their wages to be tripled, while the wages of the workers in the supply chain were doubled.

This overview leads us to conclude that in managing the health emergency China has provided a universal service of access to medical care that capitalist countries, in some cases, fail to provide.

Not only China but other socialist countries have also been able to meet the COVID-19 challenge, protecting the population from the spread of the pandemic.

II. Two models in comparison

In the world, two antithetical approaches have been adopted in the fight against COVID-19: the Chinese method (adopted throughout Asia) based on the suppression of the virus through the elimination of its spread, and the Western method, based on "flock immunity," which therefore allows the virus to spread with a control over its speed of propagation. The two models mentioned above are the result of two opposing approaches to the economic and production spheres. In the first case the priority is identified in the mission of saving human lives, before anything else. Therefore, the temporary closure of non-essential economic activities is considered acceptable. In the second case, the death of hundreds of thousands of people is accepted as a necessary natural fact, in order to allow the "natural" performance of private economic activities and therefore to be able to still generate profits and revenues.

In the countries for which the flock immunity strategy has been most widely applied, we can find the United States and Great Britain. Comparing the speeches of the political leaders of these countries with those of China, it emerges that China's approach was the only one that places man at the centre of political initiative. In mid-February 2020, the Chinese President declared that "doing a good job in preventing and controlling the epidemic situation is directly related to the safety of people's lives and health, and directly related to overall economic and social stability, as well as to China's openness. (...) It is necessary to coordinate the deployment of personnel as much as possible, to gather as many elite soldiers and seriously ill patients as possible, to carry out unified treatment and to fight to reduce mortality."[1] Weeks later, and despite WHO warnings about the danger of this new coronavirus, the US president denied the existence of the problem, while the British premier stressed that the virus should not be stopped.[2]

It is precisely the Chinese socialist system and the characteristics of its government that have made it possible to include the fight against the virus and the needs of its citizens as the top non-negotiable priority of its action, mobilising all national resources for this purpose. The long lockdown has made

---

1   Xi Jinping, "Speech at the meeting of the Standing Committee of the Political Bureau of the CPC Central Committee during the study of the response to the new coronavirus pneumonia epidemic," *Qiushi*, February 15, 2020, http://www.qstheory.cn/dukan/qs/2020-02/15/c_1125572832.htm.
2   D. Trump: "We have it under control. It's-going to be just fine" ("President Donald Trump sits down with CNBC's Joe Kernen at the WEF in Davos," CNBC, January 22, 2020, https://www.cnbc.com/2020/01/22/cnbc-transcript-president-donald-trump-sits-down-with-cnbcs-joe-kernen-at-the-world-economic-forum-in-davos-switzerland.html); D. Cameron: "One of the theories is perhaps you could take it on the chin, take it all in one go and allow the disease to move through the population without really taking as many draconian measures. I think we need to strike a balance" (BBC, UK moving towards 'delay' phase of virus plan as cases hit 115, March 5, 2020, https://www.bbc.com/news/uk-51749352).

a decisive contribution to the isolation of viral outbreaks and has activated a virtuous social circle able to drive citizens to adopt responsible conduct; and doing so has minimised social contacts and the spread of epidemics. This aspect has not been found in capitalist countries. In southern European countries (such as Italy), for example, governments have not been able to maintain the policy of freezing economic activities due to strong pressure exercised by economic forces (independent and actually constraining political power) and the political conflict between the states and, within them, between local authorities and central government and among political forces.

The virus (and the consequent actions to stop any production) has had a different impact on the European and Chinese population. In the last ten years real salaries in China have more than doubled and, the welfare state has increased significantly. The number of hospital beds per 1,000 people (4.34) is significantly higher than the Organization for Economic Co-operation and Development (OECD) average (2.9), the US (2.7) and the UK (2.5) and this has clearly affected China's ability to minimise the hardship caused by the epidemic.[1]

Conversely, the working classes in Europe and the US have suffered a harsh policy for neoliberal austerity in the last decade, with drastic cuts in health and social services, which has made the COVID-19 mortality rate high.

Even during this coronavirus emergency, the social impact on the working classes in capitalist countries has been very high: there has been an increase in unemployment and difficulties in sustaining a growing number of families. The Communist Party of China (CPC), on the other hand, accompanied the closure of production facilities with income support for workers, for example by putting mortgage and credit card payments on standby and providing subsidies to ensure that salaries would continue to be paid, or providing logistical assistance in

---

1   "List of Countries by Hospital Beds," see https://en.wikipedia.org/wiki/List_of_countries_by_hospital_beds.

receiving food and drugs to people in isolation.

One of the keys to China's success proved to be the existence of a powerful and structured Communist Party, capable of a widespread presence in all districts and workplaces and ensuring that people's basic needs were met. Such an aspect, once again, breaks with the dominant interpretation of the information system in Western countries, which describes the CPC as an ankylosed and bureaucratic party, even it is not about to collapse. While in mature capitalist countries the management of the emergency has faced a disarticulation of political power (for example, in the USA each state has developed its own policies of social distancing, generating disinformation about the real risks of the virus and a very fragmented political response), the Chinese socialist system has allowed a unified action in the whole country and municipalities to fight the epidemic and protect the population.

III. The Western response and the Italian case

Despite the very high level of deaths from COVID-19 registered in its own country, the US Administration is focused on building real economic and financial reprisals against Beijing. Just as the whole world watched in dismay at the images of mass graves for the deaths from COVID-19 in New York (images that we would expect to see in the poor suburbs of the world), Trump and his staff have long pressured the intelligence services to find the "evidence" of Chinese responsibility in order to fuel a new Sino-American challenge expressly wanted by the White House[1] (this was what the Washington Post candidly talked about in those weeks).

In fact, it is based on the idea of removing – wholly or partially – the sovereign immunity from China, which is guaranteed by law to countries, in order to give legal actions and claims for damages a chance of success. However, it cannot be

---

1 "U.S. officials crafting retaliatory actions against China over coronavirus as President Trump fumes," *The Washington Post*, April 30, 2020, see https://www.washingtonpost.com/business/2020/04/30/trump-china-coronavirus-retaliation/.

ruled out that the US Administration is in fact already considering new trade tariffs: according to press reports, Trump and some of his staff have been discussing the imposition of sanctions worth $1 trillion on future Chinese imports to make up for the coronavirus damage.

The same Chinese solidarity campaign, thanks to which medical staff and medical equipment arrived in the countries affected by the virus, was an opportunity for the Western media to incite controversy and insinuate that behind the donation of aid there was the intention from Beijing (but also from Moscow and Havana) to increase its influence in some key countries in the NATO area, exploiting the congenital divisions of the European Union.

What those media do not say is that the EU is already deeply divided and shaken by the economic crisis that started in 2007, the migration crisis since 2015, Brexit and the inability to build solidarity and aid policies between member states. What is condemning the EU to division and marginality, and what is condemning the economies of southern European countries, is not the Chinese proposal to establish and strengthen the Silk Road of Health, but the firm position of Germany, Austria and the Netherlands to persevere with the austerity policy and prevent the European Central Bank (ECB) from financing public spending or accepting the principle of "shared European debt." The EU is in crisis because of the congenital rules inscribed in its founding Treaties and the unbalanced relations between its member states. The possibility of cooperation with China, if anything, represents a political opportunity for some of its member states not to be crushed by the burden of debt that the European mechanism itself has inflicted.

It is quite clear that these campaigns have the clear aim of building a galvanised international public opinion in the fight against a common enemy which, instead of being the virus, is identified in socialist China, in its process of economic rise and in its effective governance which is increasingly evident at a global stage. Just as the ideological (and political, military and economic) mobilization against the incumbent threat posed by the Soviet Union represented a cement in the Western capitalist world after the Second World War, today the mobilization against China and the Chinese Communist Party represents an attempt to build a new broad anti-communist alliance, whose main enemy is the People's Republic of China and the emergence of a bloc of countries that have not adopted the practices of the Washington Consensus, or an attempt to keep countries that give to China a political legitimacy within this alliance that Washington would like to prevent it. And this is the case in Italy.

At first it was evident that the international campaign to claim compensation from China for the damage committed by COVID-19 had also taken place in Italy. The (modest, but paradigmatic) signal was given by the small case of the Hotel De La Poste in Cortina d'Ampezzo, which sued the Ministry of Health of the People's Republic of China in the Court of Belluno for damages. More significant, on the other hand, was the case of the Lombardy Region's request (the region that first and foremost received the help of Chinese medical experts in Italy) for "compensation" of 20 billion euros from Beijing for the consequences of COVID-19.[1] This request is driven by the party that governs the region and that was a member of the government when Italy signed the Memorandum of Understanding (MOU) with China over the Belt and Road Initiative (BIS), and whose Secretary-General declares now that Europe must "ask Beijing for money. We all know where the virus started." And it is also indicative that Paolo Mieli, from the pages of the most important national daily newspaper, pointed out that "for the first time in many years the Western countries' front has reassembled itself in asking China for clarification on how COVID-19 was born and then it has spread, (...) however, to reflect the fact that Italy is the only country in the world to have welcomed half a million masks sent (for a fee) from China with a truly excessive jubilation."[2]

---

1 Adnkronos, "Lega: 'Lombardia chiederà 20 miliardi di danni alla Cina'," April 29, 2020, see https://www.adnkronos.com/fatti/politica/2020/04/29/lega-lombardia-chiedera-miliardi-danni-alla-cina_HTO6WCnZXEjrGlpJRuspGl.html?refresh_ce.
2 Paolo Mieli, "Sulla Cina troppe ambiguità," April 26, 2020, see https://www.corriere.it/editoriali/20_aprile_26/sulla-cina-troppe-ambiguita-5b11beb8-87e9-11ea-8a3a-5c7a635a608c.shtml.

Why is this happening? Because there is a capitalist reorganization project in progress that aims to prevent the contradictions of capitalist countries, from leading to a reversal of power relations at an international level. Italy, which is a key component in the Atlantic camp for its relations with China, especially in the BIS and 5G dossiers, is now under lot of scrutiny.

This project of capitalist reorganisation moves along two lines: a strong domestic repression and reduction of the working classes' rights and a foreign strategy aimed at preventing the Italian government from giving China the political legitimacy it deserves. The Atlantic (and EU) line is clear in this regard: economic and trade relations are allowed, but it is forbidden to concede political equality to a country led by the Communist Party which remains, according to Emmanuel Macron's definition, a "systemic competitor." It is with this consciousness that we should look at what happened in Italy in recent months when, in the midst of a health emergency, a capitalist restructuring project took shape with a change in the board of directors of the most important trade association of Italian industry and in the proprietary structure of the largest publishing group which, with considerable violence, immediately changed all the editors of the controlled newspapers, imposing distinctly pro-Atlantic people. These changes highlight the emergence of a new transversal and powerful "anti-Chinese party" which, with its representatives in the private sector, the media and politics, is trying to prevent a change in the orientation of Italian public opinion in favour of Beijing. The warning signals were sounded by a number of polls and sentiment analysis carried out in the middle of a pandemic. The results of these analyses are very interesting and instructive.

After the arrival of Chinese (March 13, 2020) and Russian (March 22, 2020) aid, a study of Google search engine results and the trend in citation volumes on Social and Digital Media demonstrated that Italian interest in China and Russia was immeasurably greater than the announcement of US and EU aid.

The Sentiment Analysis shows that "over 97.7k citations for 'Chinese aid' between 1st and 31st March. Positive sentiment exceeds negative sentiment (27% vs.

19.8% respectively): the trend of volumes over time clearly shows how the arrival of aid is immediately described and welcomed with great positivity (peaks on 13th-15th March)." Finally, "the semantic analysis of the words most frequently associated with Sentiment Analysis shows significant examples from the contents analysed: negative sentiment is mainly connected to the domestic political debate, to the relations with the European Union and NATO and only partially are allegations against China."[1]

Also the report of the Munich Security Conference, a Bavarian military and diplomatic gathering, records an attitude of Italy's openness to Russia and China: out of 100 interviewed in case of conflict between the USA and Russia and in case of conflict between the USA and China, Italy is the country in Europe where the percentage of those who would take sides for the two Eurasian countries is the highest.[2] But the most sensational result, also because it was broadcast on all national TVs, was that of two surveys conducted by the SWG demoscopic institute. The first survey, carried out on the March 25-27, 2020, questioned the sample which countries in terms of foreign policy, economy and diplomatic relations were the best friend states and which ones were the enemy states of Italy. Incredibly, among the states friends, the survey sample indicated China, Russia and only later on, their historical ally, the United States of America. Germany, France and the United Kingdom (United States in fourth place) were among the countries considered enemies, i.e. the countries that most of all were perceived as those who opposed forms of aid to Italy which, in those days, was the country most affected by COVID-19.

The second survey, carried out between 1st and 3rd April 2020, questioned the sample on which countries outside the EU, Italy should look more carefully

---

1 Gabriele Iacovino, Marco Di Liddo e Filippo Tansini, "Incertezze e Supremazia Informativa: l'Ecosistema Italia di Fronte alla Pandemia," Centro Studi Internazionali, Aprile 2020, pp. 6-8.
2 Out of 100 interviewees, 65% want to opt for neutrality in the event of conflict between the USA and Russia, 9% do not know, 17 are on the side of the USA and 9the highest figure among European countrieswith Russia. In the event of a US-China conflict, 63 declare themselves neutral, 10 say they do not know, 20 are on the US side and 7once again the highest number among European countrieswith China. Taken from: Munich Security Report 2020, p. 19.

to develop its international alliances. 36% of the sample indicated China, while 30% indicated the United States. Aggregating these data along the axis of political affiliations, we find that the United States is seen with greater interest by centre-right voters (51%), while Democratic Party voters look to China (45%). The voters most open to Beijing are those of the 5 Star Movement (53%).

IV. Conclusion

Precisely for the reasons listed above, in the eyes of large populations around the world, the emergency management generated by COVID-19 has made clear the differences between the way adopted by capitalist countries, oriented towards the defence of private profit in spite of the health and life of their citizens, and that of socialist China, which has placed human life at the centre of its initiative. Not only that: Chinese management has proved more effective and, for the first time in many years, has begun to be seen as a practicable model even in countries traditionally linked to the Atlantic alliance and the capitalist system. These are the reasons that explain the hard counter-offensive of the last few weeks, led by the USA, which is at the forefront of an anti-Chinese (and anti-communist) coalition in all countries.

This article is dedicated to Chinese doctors who came to Italy to help the population affected by the virus with their experience and knowledge accumulated on the grassroots in the battle of Wuhan against COVID-19, I dedicated to Chinese citizens living abroad who were discriminated and were victims of Sino-phobia; to all those who lost a relative due to this epidemic. COVID-19 is a common enemy of humanity and all mankind, without distinction of races and countries, is called to face it together. We are not only a part of this world, but a community with a shared future for all mankind.

The Crisis of COVID-19 Pandemic Reveals the Fundamental Weaknesses of the Capitalist System

[Japan] Onishi Hiroshi

Edited by Zhu Xuxu[1]   *Translated by Li Yi   Finalized by He Jun*

About the Author

Onishi Hiroshi, male, was born in Kyoto in 1956. He is a professor of the Faculty of Economics at Keio University, a professor emeritus of Kyoto University, and has a PhD degree in economics. The posts he assumes include: vice-chairman of Japan-China Friendship Association, deputy director of World Association for Political Economy, former president of the Japan Association for Northeast Asia Regional Studies, executive member of the Affairs Bureau of Socialist Theories Society, former chairman of the Executive Council of Basic Economic Science Research Institute, member of the Council of The Japan Association for Modern China Studies, and executive member of the Council of the International Association for Asian Community Studies. His main research fields include political economy (theory of optimal economic growth in Marxist economics), statistics, issues on politics and economy of modern China, and issues on East Asian economies.

---

1   Zhu Xuxu, doctoral candidate at School of Marxism, Graduate School of Chinese Academy of Social Sciences.

Abstract

Since the outbreak of COVID-19, there have been heated discussions on the relationship between state systems and anti-pandemic effectiveness in many countries around the world. With capitalist countries as the research objects during this pandemic, this paper, through discussing the relationship between state systems and crisis handling capabilities and effectiveness, reveals the fundamental weaknesses of capitalist system in meeting the challenge, and serves as a response to public opinions in the world today. Given the escalating conflicts in capitalist countries as a result of COVID-19, it looks to the prospect of a socialist society in the future.

I. Abrupt changes in the public opinions on COVID-19

When COVID-19 was beginning to spread around the world, the international public opinion led by the Western World stigmatized China by criticizing its slow response and "autocratic system." However, such international public opinion has made an about-face completely after China effectively put the domestic epidemic situation under control and provided assistance to other countries in coordinated efforts to fight against the pandemic. This is due to the facts that the US, the most vociferous criticizer of China, has the largest number of infected cases, and that the numbers of infected cases and fatalities are increasing sharply in less populated countries in Europe.

In fact, the prevention and control measures against the COVID-19 pandemic differ greatly from country to country and from region to region. In Germany, where the government strictly requires that nucleic acid testing (NAT) be conducted, the fatality rate is much lower than that of other countries despite the sharp increase in infected cases. In South Korea, "public health doctors" under the administration of the state were immediately sent to all parts of the country after the outbreak of the COVID-19 epidemic, and nucleic acid tests were conducted on a large scale.

In China, the construction of hospitals that admit and treat COVID-19 patients was completed within 10 days in the city of Wuhan, which was locked down. Moreover, the government further intensifies the management of citizens' personal health information through employing health QR code in mobile apps.

II. The policies adopted in preventing and controlling the COVID-19 pandemic should not be used as the criterion for judging a state system

At present, the policies adopted in responding to the COVID-19 pandemic vary greatly from country to country. It is incredibly unthinkable for Western countries to use the policies of epidemic prevention and control as a criterion for judging whether a social system is "autocratic" or not. Yuval Noah Harari, a world-renowned historian, is a representative of this opinion. On April 3, 2020, *Nihon Keizai Shimbun*[1] also divided countries into four types based on the degree of constraints on people's freedom of movements in the course of epidemic prevention. By a sequence based on the intensity of the measures adopted, the country implementing the toughest measures is China, followed by France, Italy, Spain, Britain, Germany, the US, Japan and other countries. As a matter of fact, these reports represent an ideological struggle deliberately launched by Western countries in a bid to prevent China from becoming a world leader, although they have learned from China's experience in the fight against the epidemic.

At present, the Western countries' understanding of the prevention and control measures of various countries completely goes against the facts. Kenji Shibuya, senior advisor to the World Health Organization (WHO) and professor of King's College London, stressed that it was essential to conduct nucleic acid tests and keep people in quarantine or isolation as much as possible in order to stem the

---

1   Hiroyuki Akita, "Japan Cannot Afford to Lose in Responding to Coronavirus," *Nihon Keizai Shimbun*, April 3, 2020.

spread of COVID-19. In East Asia, the Chinese government sent a 40,000-strong medical team to help the lockdown city of Wuhan, and South Korea also conducted strict nucleic acid testing. These measures are essentially different from Japan's measures of deliberately restricting the nucleic acid testing to prevent and conceal the increases in the infected cases. It is reported that citizens of China, Japan and South Korea have developed immunity against COVID-19 after they are inoculated with BCG vaccine, and it is therefore mistakenly believed that they have stronger immunity against COVID-19 than citizens in European countries and the US. However, the main reason for the smaller number of infected cases in Japan is that the Japanese government deliberately restricts people to undergo nucleic acid testing. Some estimates point out that the infected cases in Japan will probably exceed those in European countries. In Japan there were even people dying from COVID-19 while waiting for government permission to get nucleic acid testing. Under such circumstances, people infected with the coronavirus who were not given testing or treatment in a timely manner appear in large numbers on the street or in hospitals in Japan. For instance, among the patients coming to the hospital affiliated with Keio University where I work, about six percent are infected cases. This situation paralyzes the medical treatment system in the hospital. At present, the efforts to prevent and control the epidemic are far from satisfactory in the US, and Japan is the least effective in the fight against the epidemic among all East Asian countries. The measures and policies adopted by the US and Japanese governments against COVID-19 are indeed worrisome.

III. Insufficiencies and defects in Japan's efforts to prevent and control the COVID-19 epidemic

In its efforts to prevent and control COVID-19, Japan not only ignores nucleic acid testing but also fails to give special attention to quarantine. For instance, in

March and April 2020, a freelance writer[1] who had home isolation experiences in both Japan and South Korea pointed out in his blog that the Japanese government was perfunctory towards home isolation. The Japanese government stipulated that starting from March 5, 2020, upon their entry into Japan, those coming from China and South Korea should go to the places designated by the Japanese government for quarantine for 14 days. However, when he entered Japan at Narita Airport on March 28, 2020, the airport staff members did not conduct testing on him at all; instead, they merely gave him a health survey form. The "14-day home isolation" was just an oral requirement without any compulsory measures applied for implementation. Two weeks later, the freelance writer left Japan for South Korea through Narita Airport. This shows that Japanese residents can leave their own houses without restriction and the government completely ignores home isolation. The Japanese government prohibits passengers from using public transport on their way from Narita Airport to their homes. However, a passenger is allowed to leave the airport so long as he/she can tell the airport staff that he/she would be picked up by a family member. Moreover, a friend said that when taxis are the only choice, only the wealthy can afford it. How can people living in Hokkaido or northeastern Japan get home from Narita Airport if they are not allowed to use the public transport? In other words, the Japanese government shirks its duty by irresponsibly formulating ineffective policies on prevention and control of the the COVID-19 epidemic.[2]

In comparison, South Korea adopts more proactive and effective measures against the epidemic. According to the same freelance writer, on the one hand, flight attendants on the planes from Japan to South Korea would distribute "Instructions on Smart Home Diagnosis Guide Application" to passengers. Upon their arrival

---

1   Narigawa Aya, "Thoughts About the Experiences of Home Isolation in Japan and South Korea Where Coronavirus Spreads," April 28, 2020, see: https://globe.asahi.com/article/13299164.

2   In fact, the "dramatic increase" in the number of COVID-19 patients was caused by the failure to effectively control the "second wave of virus" from European countries and the US. According to the son of a friend, upon his entry from Finland to Japan at Narita Airport during the epidemic, he was not restricted by any measures against the coronavirus at all.

in South Korea, passengers are required to download and register this app on their mobile phones and fill their home address in details and report their body temperatures twice a day. If a passenger lives in the city proper of Seoul, he/she is required to undergo an on-the-spot nucleic acid test. If the passenger does not show any syndrome of COVID-19, he/she is directed to the designated place to go into isolation free of charge. On the other hand, the South Korean government provides special-purpose buses and taxies for those leaving the airport for their homes. Any person entering South Korea should strictly observe the stipulations concerning home isolation, and violators of these stipulations will be fined. The government would distribute disinfectant solutions, face masks, food and other anti-epidemic supplies and grant living subsidies and paid vacations (from other sources of information) to those observing the stipulations. Moreover, the government would conduct nucleic acid testing on a person on the 13th day after he/she enters South Korea to see to it that the person is not infected with the virus (from other sources of information) before the 14-day home isolation can be lifted. These are the compulsory measures adopted by South Korea to ensure effective isolation.

China has designated hotels for those entering its territory to go into isolation. In Tianjin and Nanjing, one will be asked to take a body temperature once he/she goes outdoors. In supermarkets entries and exits are clearly marked to prevent cross-infection.

In summary, South Korea and China adopt highly responsible prevention and control measures led by the government. In contrast, the Japanese government adopts the strategy of "trying not to come into contact with anybody," which is extremely irresponsible and only serves to cause panic among the public.

IV. Given the severe challenge posed by COVID-19, the different measures adopted by China and Japan toward businesses manifest the strengths of China's socialist system

As countries adopted very different measures in their response to the epidemic, it is extremely absurd for the Western countries to generalize such differences as the differences between two state systems – the "autocratic" system and the "democratic" system. For instance, in South Korea, the most "democratic" political force still has to rely on "autocracy" to obtain positive anti-epidemic results.

Today, in *Nanjing's Anti-epidemic Scene,*[1] a short documentary made by the Japanese Director Takeuchi Ryo that has proved to be very popular among Japanese and Chinese netizens, it is reported that Nanjing citizens willingly provide the government with detailed travel information, such as the time, the place, the train or subway they take, and the final destinations. Such information is essential for China to do a good job in preventing and controlling COVID-19. In the era of the Internet, it is convenient for citizens to report their travel information through smart phones and special apps. Their willingness to give this information to the government is indication that they trust the government.[2] The Western countries' clamor about ordinary people in China suffering from rigorous control imposed by the government goes against the truth. In fact, citizens collaborate with the government in the fight against the epidemic by providing their travel information of their own accord.

The prevention and control measures adopted by the Chinese government are effective in managing citizens as well as businesses. In my opinion, this is an important distinction between China and Japan in terms of epidemic prevention and control. By the beginning of April, 2020, large numbers of workers in Japan still had to commute to and from work in packed trains every day. Even after the government

---

1 "The Japanese Living in China – A Documentary Directed by Takeuchi Ryo," April 23, 2020, see: https://creators.yahoo.co.jp/takeuchiryo/0200056742.

2 According to the findings of The 2018 Edelman Trust Barometer conducted in 28 countries by Edelman Public Relations Worldwide, China was the country with the largest number of people having "trust in government" (84 percent). According to the findings of an Ipsos Poll conducted in 2019, China was the country with the highest proportion of respondents having trust in the government of their own country (94 percent). In their book entitled *China, a Happy Country Subject to Monitoring* (NHK), Kajitani Kai and Kota Takaguchi made an intensive study on the degree of trust of the Chinese nationals on their government. Their findings are also useful as reference.

had demanded that "contact between people be restricted," almost half of the workers had to commute by trains.[1] No detailed information about personal use of the means of public transport is collected, as what was done in Nanjing, China, let alone the "prevention of cross-infection." To avoid direct contact, Japanese people voluntarily restrict their visits to relatives and friends or travels during the May Day golden week, and reduced the frequency of dining out with their friends and family members. All activities organized by the academic societies and the Japan-China Friendship Association with which I am affiliated are canceled. However, Japanese enterprises continue their production. I believe the imbalance in the responsibilities respectively undertaken by the government and citizens is the biggest problem in the present epidemic prevention in Japan.

In modern society, the working class is essentially distinct from slaves as follows: For the working class, except for the working time sold to capitalists, the remainder of the time is at their disposal. However, during the period of epidemic control, the capitalists in Japan appeal to workers to "work hard on work days and stand by (go into isolation) at home at weekends," continuing their exploitations without restrictions and depriving the working class of their freedom. Large numbers of working people are mercilessly deprived of what is left of their free time – weekends and after-work hours.

However, Chinese enterprises are totally different from their Japanese counterparts in responding to the coronavirus. According to *Japan-China Friendship Newspaper*[2] of April 25, 2020, after the vehicle component enterprises in Tianjin Economic-Technological Development Area resumed their production, they disinfected the buses that take workers to and from work, as well as offices and business premises, and isolated the workers returning from outside of Tianjin. To

---

1   DOCOMO Insight Marketing, "Survey Results of Population Statistics Based on Mobile Network," *Nihon Keizai Shimbun*, April 28, 2020.
2   "New Coronavirus: Domestic Life in China Today," *Japan-China Friendship Newspaper*, April 25, 2020.

avoid direct contact among people during the working hours, factories demanded
that workers keep a distance of at least 1.5 meters from each other. There are
specific provisions prohibiting the use of elevators, wearing face masks and washing
hands frequently. The government also demanded that workers have their body
temperatures taken three times a day and report it to the authorities. In the report
about Nanjing it also said that enterprises have the duty of purchasing non-contact
thermometers for workers and ask them to take their body temperatures several
times a day. In Japan, however, it is almost inconceivable for the government to
exercise this type of management and control over businesses.

As to prevention and control of COVID-19, I pay more attention to how China
and Japan differ from each other concerning the management and control over the
production activities of enterprises. In China, both enterprises and individuals are
required to undertake corresponding responsibilities, while in Japan, individuals are
required to restrict their activities but enterprises are not subject to such restrictions.
This is the concrete embodiment of the differences between the socialist system and
the capitalist system in terms of epidemic control. To limit individuals' activities,
the Japanese government issued Emergency Declaration, and subsequently imposed
some restrictions on KTVs, slot machine shops, bars,[1] beauty parlors, indoor
stadiums, cinemas and concerts. These measures inevitably impeded the businesses
in relevant industries. In the final analysis, however, they are but an extension of
the government's policy of "restricting individuals' activities," rather than regarding
enterprises as the objects of epidemic prevention and control from the outset.

In addition, the demand that the Japanese workers suspected to have been
infected with the virus should stay home for quarantine gradually evolves into
the requirement that "do not apply for a leave of absence on account of a cold."
To carry out this measure, pharmacists in Japan kept a large amount of cold cure

---

1   In fact, Japanese bars for ordinary consumers are forced to shut down while high-end
restaurants for politicians or government officials in Akasaka are still in operation. This situation
touches upon the "issue of class" to be discussed below.

in their stores. The asymptomatic patients among workers who go to work would be rebuked by their leaders for not staying at home. Such selfish acts of Japanese capitalists during epidemic control are not feasible, and to some extent reflect the exploitative nature of the capitalist system.

V. Defects of the capitalist system as revealed because of the strike of COVID-19

From the perspective of institutional comparison, after the outbreak of COVID-19, the number of infected cases in Singapore, where no "autocratic system" is practiced, was sharply increasing, while the number of infected cases in the US surpassed one million. The increase in numbers fully reveals the defects of the capitalist system. Although the Singaporean government implemented policies to restrict cross-infection among its nationals, the situation was almost out of control when the number of infected people constantly increased as a result of a case where some 10 migrant workers shared one room. In the United States, poor people, who have been excluded from the country's medical system and who have to keep working despite the seriousness of the epidemic, are the fundamental reason why the epidemic spread rapidly in the US. These cases also demonstrate that "social system" is the fundamental factor determining the effectiveness of epidemic prevention and control.

Compared with Singapore and the US, the State of Kerala in India has been effective in the prevention and control of COVID-19. Although the first cases of infection in India were found in Kerala, this state, boasting the most equitable and complete medical system in India, quickly stemmed the spread of the virus. This result is attributed to the Communist Party of India (Marxism) which has ruled the State of Kerala over a long period of time.

Following the outbreak of COVID-19, some mainstream economists began to talk about the possibility that "Capitalism ...has to give way to the prepared socialism at least for the time being."[1] In face of the present crisis, we need to think hard about the social system itself rather than various kinds of epidemic prevention and control policies.

Moreover, the current crisis also demands that the working class have a clear sense of its own rights, and dare to stand up for them. For instance, all countries ask their citizens to refrain from going out, but the consequences for people of different classes are extremely different. It is highly unequal for owners of large houses attached with courtyards and the working people living in apartment buildings who have no place to go except for parks and libraries to observe the same stipulation of "restricting the opportunities of going outdoors" for epidemic prevention and control. Furthermore, those who have constant streams of money coming in without having to work form a sharp contrast with irregularly employed workers who will immediately lose their incomes if they resign their jobs. Here the requirement in capitalist countries that people "exercise self-control over going out" is "against the working class." In fact, personages from the mainstream society of Latin American countries have expressed the same point of view. Similar views were expressed by the prime minister of Pakistan: "If a city is locked down, the people will be saved from the COVID-19 crisis; on the other hand, some people will starve to death because of the lockdown."[2] It is known to all that the COVID-19 crisis cannot be completely resolved in the entire world so long as COVID-19 is not completely resolved among poor people and in poor countries. Therefore, it is essential that all

---

1   Willem H. Buiter, "Socialist Economy Caused by the Crisis," *Nihon Keizai Shimbun*, April 23, 2020.
2   "New Coronavirus: Crisis of Making a Living Among 1.6 Billion Working People Worldwide, ILO Forecast," April 8, 2020, see: https://www.nikkei.com/article/DGXMZO58624870Z20C20A4FF8000/.

countries should strengthen their collaboration in tackling this crisis.[1]

VI. Prospects for Communism under the background of the COVID-19 pandemic

Against the backdrop of globalization, the key problem that has to be addressed in the present-day world is to contain the spread of COVID-19 in impoverished countries, which has also become the focus of concern of all countries. There are two main viewpoints on epidemic control in impoverished countries: The first viewpoint holds that the impoverished people and countries are forced to embark on the path of "herd immunity" as they are incapable of implementing any effective control measures. Subsequently, other countries will follow suit. The second viewpoint is that the problems faced by impoverished countries should be regarded as the problems of our own, that other countries should provide medical assistance to them and work together with them to win final victory against the epidemic. Initially, Britain adopted the policy of "herd immunity"; so did Sweden, which later proclaimed its victory. Although it is quite reasonable in adopting this strategy, we should be aware that Sweden's success is based on the fact that the country has few really poor people and a sound medical system. In other words, the Swedish experience of fighting against the epidemic is not relevant to impoverished countries. In addition, it is fair and reasonable for all countries to close their national boundaries and cities for a period of time before the infectious power of COVID-19

---

1   Although the difficulties of Japan in response to the crisis are not discussed here, the behaviors of American troops stationed in Japan, which are out of control of the Japanese government, cause great troubles to anti-epidemic efforts in Japan. For instance, when infected cases were reported on USS Ronald Reagan CVN-76 which sat anchored at Yokosuka, the Japanese government could not adopt any restrictive measures against any activities of these people in Japan. According to the stipulations on their "privileges in Japan," the American soldiers can enter the territory of Japan without passports and their freedom of movement is protected. The crux of this problem lies in Japan's subordination to the US.

is figured out and the relevant statistics about immunity is available. Given the current situation, the second viewpoint of strengthening international coordination and support is highly necessary. After China successfully kept the epidemic under control through city lockdowns, it began to promote its experience worldwide under the slogan of "building a healthy Silk Road." Its efforts should be recognized.

On top of the strengthened international collaboration, mutual assistance between nationals of different countries will be intensified as well. In response to the coronavirus, the Chinese people are united and ready to provide mutual assistance, which is worthy of note. For instance, after Wuhan announced the lockdown, the Chinese government sent more than 40,000 medical workers to aid the local people. To assist these medical workers, a dairy producer in Shanghai provided them with the materials that can lessen the harm to their ears when they wear face masks. Fudan University provided the children of these medical workers with volunteer online services for helping the children in their studies. An airline in the Inner Mongolia Autonomous Region decided to grant the medical workers dispatched to Wuhan three-year free access to the first-class lounges at 20 airports under its jurisdiction. People wrote letters of thanks to encourage the medical workers giving assistance in Wuhan. In Shanghai, volunteers expressed support to hospitals specially providing treatment for COVID-19 patients, and helped those observing self-quarantine at home do shopping and throw away rubbish, and distributed face masks to them.[1] Isn't it the communist society that is pursued by Marxism? The well-being of residents is not improved by relying on the participation through the

---

1   These cases are provided by Professor Zhu Jianrong from Toyo Gakuen University. Apart from the cases cited in the text, the online medical service enterprises in China which have offered medical services free of charge perform well in epidemic prevention and control. These enterprises include Jingdong Health under the banner of Jingdong Group, Ali Health under the banner of Alibaba Group, and Tencent Healthcare under the banner of Tencent Group. Although they provide paid medical services afterwards for the purpose of making profits, corporate social responsibility has become the prerequisite and basis of the sustained development of such online medical service enterprises in case of emergency in China. Performing such responsibility is of important significance.

use of compulsory force by the state, but through the mutual assistance network system spontaneously developed by non-government sectors. This is the essence of the communist society that is pursued by Marxism.

In Japan, workers stay at home to work online as COVID-19 has yet to be contained. This way of working is becoming ever more popular. The mode of work whereby workers are always subject to monitoring by their supervisors is gradually shifting to one whereby workers exercise self-management over their own working. This is an important issue that is worth pondering over during the post-capitalist era. The entire world is talking about thorough changes in the world structure following the end of the pandemic. The voices of "transcending capitalism and entering socialism" raised by Marxist economists are louder than before.

Strategy on the COVID-19 Pandemic

[America] Luis Suarez-Villa

Edited by Gao Jingyu[1]

About the Author

Prof. Suarez-Villa has been a faculty member of the University of California since 1982, and was a co-founder of the Department of Planning, Policy and Design. Luis Suarez-Villa specializes in the study of corporate capitalism, technology, innovation, and international development from the perspective of critical political economy and social analysis. He is fluent in five languages, and has traveled to 69 nations around the world in relation to his academic work. His most recent book, *Corporate Power, Oligopolies, and the Crisis of the State* (Albany: State University of New York Press, 2015), explores the rising influence of oligopolistic corporations in contemporary society. Two previous books, *Technocapitalism: A Critical Perspective on Technological Innovation and Corporatism* (Philadelphia: Temple University Press, 2009) and *Globalization and Technocapitalism: The Political Economy of Corporate Power and Technological Domination* (London: Ashgate, 2012), explore the emergence of a new, twenty-first century version of capitalism grounded in technology and science, and the political economy of corporate power and influence associated with it.

---

1 Gao Jingyu, assistant research fellow of the Academy of Marxism, Chinese Academy of Social Sciences.

Abstract

The COVID-19 pandemic clearly demonstrates that solving major problems affecting humanity's survival calls for solidarity around the world. Selfishness on a national scale, supremacism, chauvinism, racism and imperialism – of any kind – are deleterious to the survival of humanity on earth. World leaders who indulge in promoting views that foster such attitudes must be condemned. China is eminently placed to lead a new global configuration of power based on mutual respect, solidarity and equality. China's experience with imperialism in past centuries is very important to understand in this regard. In the face of the present pandemic, it is necessary to adopt multi-facet and multi-level actions based on global solidarity and coordination. These actions include creation of a global repository for public knowledge, reducing inequality in education, establishing a world fund and rewarding system to encourage young people to study medicine and get involved in relevant medical projects, and that China and Cuba can cooperate in setting up medical establishments and conducting training in medicine.

All events related to the pandemic demonstrate the need for solidarity around the planet. This is essential not only in regards to the control of this and any future pandemics, but also for solving major problems affecting humanity's survival – such as global warming, rising ocean levels, and the accelerating destruction of nature. The COVID-19 pandemic has, specifically, made it clear how small our planet is, and how important it is for humanity to cooperate – if we are to survive the very serious challenges that we will face in this century.

Selfishness on a national scale, supremacism, chauvinism, racism and imperialism – of any kind – are deleterious to the survival of humanity on earth. World leaders who indulge in promoting views that foster such attitudes must be condemned, and the people of all nations of the world must be made aware of the damage they cause. Rising socio-economic inequality, deepening social injustices, and the plundering of other nations' resources are among the logical consequences of such attitudes and the actions they implement. Nations and leaders that demonstrate anti-social and inhuman attitudes will inevitably face a loss of credibility and influence among the peoples of the world. It is therefore important that we advance toward a new global configuration of power based on solidarity, cooperation, and mutual trust.

China is eminently placed to lead a new global configuration of power based on mutual respect, solidarity and equality. China's experience with imperialism in past centuries is very important to understand in this regard, as it allows one to see how its current politico-economic system allowed it to overcome immense obstacles. The introduction of opium into China by imperialist interests in the nineteenth century, for example, caused immense damage to the Chinese people. It was, at the bottom, part of a ploy to force China to submit to exploitation and to the plunder of its resources. The opium wars are said to have caused tens of millions of deaths through combat, mutilation, addiction and disease, and their effects were felt by several subsequent generations of Chinese. The world must not forget this horrible tragedy, and no effort should be spared to ensure that it cannot be repeated.

The COVID-19 pandemic, in particular, has made very clear the need for global coordination and cooperation in treating all aspects of health and disease. In the case of any epidemic – and even more so in the case of a pandemic – it is not enough to collect data and to inform, but to take concrete actions to save lives – actions that only global solidarity and cooperation can ensure.

One such action could be the creation of a global repository for public knowledge, of how different illnesses can spread across borders, and the sort of measures that might be pursued. This can then be codified in specific measures to be taken, and the formulation of appropriate policies on a global scale. Since contagion through human contact is obviously a major problem – as in the case of COVID-19 – it is important that everyone realize the consequences of mass contagion, and the efforts that must be pursued at both the personal and collective levels.

For this purpose, for example, dedicated channels of information on contagious diseases – in multiple languages – could be considered. This could become part of a continuous global broadcast effort operating in all time zones, 24 hours per day – via satellite – accessible for all to view, even in the most remote villages and rural areas of the planet. Conferences and seminars dedicated to the case of infectious diseases could be broadcast around the world freely, beyond any coverage of news events or circumstances that may be provided by other media. The World Health Organization is formidably placed to lead such a global information broadcast resource, as is China itself with its vast experience in health care and medicine. Diffusion of knowledge of traditional Chinese medicine could be part of such a global broadcasting operation, or it could be provided in a separate channel along with other forms of traditional medicine from around the world.

Rallying a strong force to combat pandemics and epidemics must be a multifaceted, multilevel effort that engages all the peoples of the world, and all governments. One such effort must be the reduction of inequalities in educational access and quality. Only an informed and educated population can deal with the serious problems posed by a pandemic – or any epidemic – effectively. The reduction of such inequalities in educational access is also fundamental for increasing the population of physicians and medical personnel.

For this purpose, a world fund that makes it possible for young people to study medicine and health care anywhere – in any related specialty – could be created. Because it is very expensive to establish medical schools, and educate physicians and personnel, we must remember that not all nations might be able to engage in this effort. Thus, international medical brigades composed of physicians and professionals in all health specialties, could be made available to nations that cannot afford to invest sufficient resources in medical and health-related professional education. China, with its historical experience with the barefoot-doctor program in the 1950s and 60s, and today Cuba – with its medical brigades now serving the poorest populations in over 60 nations around the world – can provide valuable knowledge on the policies that need to be considered.

Global recognition should be established to reveal and reward the efforts of those who engage in such efforts. Perhaps a prize equivalent to the Nobel – but dedicated to social medicine and the implementation of medical or health programs among the poorest populations of the world – could be created. China, because of its influence in the world, and the vast resources it can marshal, would be the ideal nation to create and to house this initiative.

The creation of a world-class university of medicine for training personnel that would engage in this effort would be another important step. China already has institutions capable of undertaking this vital objective, as does Cuba – with its Escuela Latinoamericana de Medicina (ELAM). In the case of Cuba, greater cooperation with China would be extremely beneficial. All the more so, since Cuba – with only about 11 million in population and located 90 miles from the United States – has achieved its excellence in social medicine despite brutal, multifaceted US economic and military aggression that has lasted more than half a century.

Only through a coordinated, concerted global effort can the challenges posed by the current realities of our planet be faced – whether they involve pandemics, epidemics, any collective aspect of medicine and health care. China can and should lead the way in this regard.

Cuba received about 4 million visitors in 2019. Air China has a weekly flight, Beijing to Havana. Maybe other Chinese airlines could be encouraged to fly to Cuba, and for Chinese people to visit. In social medicine, Cuba's experience could be of interest to many Chinese students. Perhaps a joint China-Cuba university could be established in Cuba, to promote China-Cuba educational relations. A school of social medicine and health care, teaching Chinese traditional medicine – among other subjects – might be highly beneficial. It would be the first such institution in Latin America. China is already the most important trading partner for most Latin American nations. Establishing such an institution could take China-Latin America relations to a new level, beyond the commercial relations.

It Is Utterly Unreasonable for the West to Blame China for COVID-19

[Spain] Xulio Ríos

Edited by Jin Chengwei[1] Li Xin[2]   Translated by Li Yi   Finalized by He Jun

---

About the Author

Xulio Ríos, born in Spain in 1958, is director of the Galician Institute of International Analysis and Documentation, director of the Chinese Policy Observatory, member of the Advisory Council of *Casa Asia*, and professor of High University Studies Institute. He has published more than 20 monographs on international issues, including *Modern China: In Rapid Development (China Moderna: Una inmersión rápida)* and *China to the Next Superpower (China, a próxima superpotencia)*.

Jin Chengwei, research fellow at the Institute of Party History and Literature of the CPC Central Committee.

2   Li Xin, doctoral candidate at the School of Marxism, Shandong University.

Abstract

This paper gives a detailed account of the outbreak and the spread of COVID-19 and the blames thrown by some Western countries on China. Based on the account, it argues why the blames are unreasonable from the perspectives of the time sequence of the pandemic, scientific research findings, and in particular, the international justice, and analyzes the Western countries' political intentions behind the blames. Finally, it discusses the trend of globalization from the perspective of the relationship between the pandemic and globalization.

I. The antagonism towards China is mounting since the outbreak of the pandemic

Some countries reiterated their criticism of China and questioned the number of infected cases in China, and the geopolitical intention of China's international aid. Such criticism comes mostly from the capitalist countries (the US, France and Britain) that were hit hard by the pandemic or the capitalist countries that normally follow the tune of hegemonism.

Now they are requesting an "independent investigation" and even "compensation" as an effort to accelerate what is known as "de-globalization," and are convinced that this can check the momentum of an irreversibly rising China. According to reports in the US, conservative research institutes and far-right organizations such as *Freedom Watch*, and public figures of the Republican Party such as Missourian senator Josh Hawley, put forward absurd advice that "the US debt to China should be cancelled." In Britain, Henry Jackson Society, a new conservative think tank, published a report entitled "Coronavirus Compensation? Assessing China's Potential Culpability and Avenues of Legal Response," which analyzed how other countries can "sue" China. Imitators have also appeared in Australia and some European countries.

II. There is no reason at all to blame China because of the pandemic

The above-mentioned "accusation" and "demand for compensation" are proposed on the ground that China "violated international law because of its failure to make known to the public the relevant information about the pandemic that broke out in Wuhan." The sequence of the pandemic shows that it is beyond doubt China did its best to respond to COVID-19 epidemic and collaborated with the World Health Organization (WHO). Stephen L. Carter, a law professor at Yale University, published an article entitled "No, China Can't Be Sued Over Coronavirus" for Bloomberg, in which he dispelled any possibility of suing China because China is subject to protection in accordance with the principle of Sovereign Immunity of State.

(I) The "accusations" to China have been refuted by research findings

The groundless accusation has been refuted by various research findings. While probing into the origin of coronavirus, scientists and experts of all categories do not rule out the possibility that the virus came from outside China. It is said that similar medical cases diagnosed with atypical virus symptoms months ago in countries like the US, Italy and Spain were probably in fact caused by the variants of coronavirus. While waiting for the scientific conclusion, it is reasonable and responsible to concentrate attention on maximizing the effect of responding to the pandemic through international collaboration.

As a matter of fact, many problems remain to be answered by scientists and health experts. We are faced with a new disease, although we sometimes deliberately do not recognize or ignore this point. We should bear in mind that the characteristics of a new virus cannot be identified and decoded at one go. As was stated by the WHO, China not only alerted the governments of other countries about the virus, but also shared all data without reserve. Given that nobody can avoid making mistakes, to date, the situation undoubtedly shows that China has delivered an overall satisfactory performance while the Western countries have performed fairly poorly on the whole.

(II) There is no legal basis for blaming China

The basis for accusing China of "intentional inaction" is said to be that China violated the stipulations of the International Health Regulation (IHR) adopted by the WHO in 2005.

First, generally speaking, judicial settlement of an international dispute is predicated on an institutional system that is agreed by the countries involved. This is the main challenge facing the settlement of any dispute through international law. The countries involved should agree that the dispute between them should be submitted to the International Court of Justice (ICJ) for settlement. They can reach agreement by adhering to the international treaty or norm that has been violated or by resorting to the decision based on a certain agreement (the special agreement reached between the countries involved on submitting the dispute for international arbitration).

It is stipulated in Article 75 of the Constitution of the WHO (Constitución de la OMS) that "Any question or dispute concerning the interpretation or application of this Constitution which is not settled by negotiation or by the Health Assembly shall be referred to the International Court of Justice..." The parties bringing the lawsuit may freely select the way of settling dispute, and may not necessarily submit the dispute to the ICJ for arbitration.

A case in point is the settlement of the armed activities on the territory of the Democratic Republic of the Congo in 2002. In accordance with Article 75 of the Constitution of the WHO, the ICJ holds that it has the right to handle any problem or dispute with respect to the interpretation and application of the Constitution of the WHO. Therefore, any dispute as to the interpretation and application of the Constitution of the WHO may be adjudicated by the ICJ in accordance with the procedure as stipulated by Article 75 of the Constitution of the WHO.

In a recent lawsuit filed by Ukraine against Russia, the ICJ interpreted Article 22 of the International Convention on the Elimination of All Forms of Racial Discrimination (Convención sobre la eliminación de todas las formas de discriminación racial), because the article stipulates the preconditions of replacing the court trial, and the application of any of these preconditions would lead to a court trial. If Article 75 of the Constitution of the WHO is interpreted as a resource of the court in handling the lawsuit filed by Ukraine against Russia, one or more countries would satisfy the conditions for negotiation, and there is no need to resort to the World Health Assembly (WHA).

The Constitution of the WHO stipulates the framework, objectives and purposes of establishing the organization; the structure, the duties and responsibilities of the organization members, yet it lacks the substantial duties and requirements of public health laws and rules. Therefore, how to file the "lawsuit" is a big challenge if a country wants to bring a "lawsuit" against China. To enter a lawsuit, a country must point out the violation against the IHR, and regard the violation as the issue or dispute related to the interpretation and application of the Constitution of the WHO.

Next, "the implementation of the International Health Regulations shall be guided by the goal of their universal application for the protection of all people of the world from the international spread of diseases." This is one of the principles contained in Article 3 of the IHR. The WHO should follow the principle of universal application of the IHR while observing the Charter of the United Nations as well as the principles of respecting the dignity, human rights and fundamental freedom of the person.

Article 5 of the IHR stipulates that "each State Party shall develop, strengthen and maintain…the capacities to detect, assess, notify and report global health emergency events."

With regard to the public health emergency of international concern, Article 6 demands that "each State Party shall notify WHO, by the most efficient means of communication available, by way of the National IHR Focal Point, and within 24 hours of assessment of public health information, of all events which may constitute a public health emergency of international concern within its territory…" China did just what was required by the stipulations.

In accordance with Article 6 of IHR, "A State Party shall…communicate to WHO…accurate and sufficiently detailed public health information available to it on the notified event, where possible including…source and type of the risk, number of cases and deaths, conditions affecting the spread of the disease and the health measures employed."

Article 7 of IHR clearly states that "if a State Party has evidence of an unexpected or unusual public health event within its territory, irrespective of origin or source, which may constitute a public health emergency of international concern, it shall provide to WHO all relevant public health information..."

In accordance with Article 37 of the Constitution of the WHO, "In the performance of their duties, the Director-General and the staff shall maintain independence and impartiality. To this end, they shall not seek or receive instructions from any government or from any authority external to the Organization. They shall refrain from any action which might reflect on their position as international officers. Each Member of the Organization on its part undertakes to respect the exclusively international character of the Director-General and the staff and not to seek to influence them."

There are two prerequisites in the "argument" of the "charge" against China. One is that the Chinese government concealed necessary information on the onset of the COVID-19 epidemic; the other is said to be that China attempted to influence the Director-General of the WHO and his team members through concealing information, providing inaccurate or false information, and providing no information at critical moment.

Then how to link the violation against the IHR with the violation against the Constitution of the WHO? It is possible to quote articles 21 and 22 of the Constitution of the WHO.

According to Article 21 of the Constitution of the WHO, "The Health Assembly shall have authority to adopt regulations concerning sanitary and quarantine requirements, nomenclatures with respect to diseases, standards with respect to diagnostic procedures for international use, and causes of death and public health practices."

According to Article 22 of the Constitution of the WHO, "Regulations adopted pursuant to Article 21 shall come into force for all Members after due notice has been given of their adoption by the Health Assembly except for such Members as may notify the Director-General of rejection or reservations within the period stated in the notice."

Therefore, it can be considered that the dispute is related to the interpretation and application of the Constitution of the WHO, or in other words, they claim that "China's violation of the IHR is an indirect violation of articles 21 and 22 of the Constitution of the WHO." But essentially, articles 21 and 22 are procedural regulations rather than substantive ones. These two articles only involve the decision-making power of the World Health Assembly and the power of the IHR to take effect, and do not impose substantial duties upon State Parties.

Next, analyze the situation of the event. Even the hypothesis that "some of China's behaviors violate the international law" is taken as the basis, what remedial measures the countries that want to "bring a lawsuit" against China are going to adopt? The International Law Commission approved the Draft Articles on Responsibility of States for International Wrongful Acts (Draft Articles) at its 53rd session held in 2001, and submitted the Draft Articles to the General Assembly of the United Nations. Although the Draft Articles have no legal binding force on any country, they enjoy relative authority and are convincing. The ICJ often uses the Draft Articles to interpret international laws and resolve the disputes between countries. The Draft Articles are strongly convincing because most of their stipulations have obtained the position of universally acknowledged customary international law.

According to Article 1 of the Draft Articles, "Every internationally wrongful act of a State entails the international responsibility of that State."

According to Article 2 of the Draft Articles, "There is an internationally wrongful act of a State when conduct consisting of an action or omission: (a) is attributable to the State under international law; and (b) constitutes a breach of an international obligation of the State."

"The conduct of any State organ shall be considered an act of that State under international law, whether the organ exercises legislative, executive, judicial or any other functions, whatever position it holds in the organization of the State, and whatever its character as an organ of the central Government or of a territorial unit of the State."

After the outbreak of COVID-19 epidemic, it is said Western politicians fabricated rumors that China intentionally or deliberately failed to perform its duty of promptly sharing the information with the WHO. As we have seen, all these accusations are not consistent with the actualities, and are baseless rumors employed to attack China.

A comprehensive interpretation of articles 12 and 14 of the Draft Articles demonstrates that "there is a breach of an international obligation by a State when an act of that State or an act having a continuing character is not in conformity with what is required of it by that obligation."

The international responsibility of a State which is entailed by an internationally wrongful act...involves legal consequences.

According to Article 31 of the Draft Articles, "The responsible State is under an obligation to make full reparation for the injury caused by the internationally wrongful act. Injury includes any damage, whether material or moral, caused by the internationally wrongful act of a State."

According to the judgment of the Corfu Channel Case delivered by the

International Court of Justice in 1949, every State has the obligation not to allow knowingly its territory to be used for acts contrary to the rights of other States.

Compensation should be made in the forms of restoring to the original state, restitution, reparation, or even guaranteeing no repetition of unlawful acts, and others. Restoring to the original state refers to that a State has the responsibility of restoring to the state prior to the committing of an unlawful act. If, under any special circumstance, it is impossible to restore to the original state or it is impossible to make sufficient compensation by restoring to the original state only, the injured State has the right to receive the reparation sufficiently indemnifying its economic loss. If neither of these two forms of compensation is satisfactory, compensation in other forms should be made to the injured State, including acknowledging the violation of law, expressing regret or making formal apology.

In summary, it is an arduous task to bring a state to face the injured states at the International Court of Justice or any other international court. As was mentioned above, the international judicial adjudication is based on reaching agreement. It is hard for China to accept the referral of the dispute to the International Court of Justice. It should not be forgotten that being a permanent member of the UN Security Council, China can exercise the right of veto when its national interests are under threat.

The decision of the International Court of Justice should be observed by parties to a dispute of their own accord. As the defender of the world peace, the UN Security Council plays a vital role in the procedures concerning the implementation of decisions by the International Court of Justice. According to Article 94 of the Charter of the United Nations, "If any party to a case fails to perform the obligations incumbent upon it under a judgment rendered by the Court, the other party may have recourse to the Security Council, which may, if it deems necessary, make recommendations or decide upon measures to be taken to give effect to the judgment." As a permanent member of the UN Security Council, China has the right to block the UN Security Council from taking any action for implementing the hypothetical verdict rendered by the International Court of Justice.

Another open and possible yet insufficiently powerful alternative is appealing to the advisory jurisdiction of the ICJ. Invoking advisory jurisdiction of the ICJ does not demand the agreement reached by all parties to the conflict. According to Article 96 of the Charter of the United Nations, "The General Assembly or the Security Council may request the International Court of Justice to give an advisory opinion on any legal question. Other organs of the United Nations and specialized agencies, which may at any time be so authorized by the General Assembly, may also request advisory opinions of the Court on legal questions arising within the scope of their activities." The problem is that the advisory opinion of the International Court of Justice lacks binding force, and the executive power of the decision is rested with the parties to the dispute and the United Nations Assembly.

III. Western countries' accusations of China are mainly out of political considerations

The weird criticisms of China heard in some countries, for instance, the US, are closely linked with the imminent presidential election to be held in November, 2020. While seeking for a second term in office, Donald Trump adopts a simple tactic of using China as a scapegoat to cover up the incompetence of the US government in responding to the public health crisis. The Republicans obviously will come up with a new platform to incorporate the views and accusations of China by the ultra-conservative right-wing forces. Anything that may distract the attention deserves a try.

Apparently the countries which increase their intensity of criticizing China because of the pandemic are keenly aware there is little legal possibility to launch any procedure of "demanding compensation." The political intention of these countries dominates the dispute, or in other words, these countries use such a tactic to cover up their incompetence in responding to this pandemic crisis, although

China has won several weeks for them with stringent control measures.

The supporters of the proposal "demanding compensation" naturally do not hope to know the responsibilities of the US in the financial crisis that broke out in 2008, nor do they hope to know that the US should make compensations for the great losses it caused in Iraq (By the way, the US made the world believe that Iraq possessed weapons of mass destruction, which was not true) and many other places.

At the regional level, China fully performs its duties and responsibilities by cooperating with the WHO in their responses to the COVID-19 pandemic. China also plays a leading role in the global response to the COVID-19 pandemic. China's donations as well as goods and materials are dispatched to all parts of the world, so do the doctors and experts from China. For a period of time, people placed their hope on the American vaccine; yet today many competitors may surpass the US in this respect. China almost solely assumes its global responsibility, although some people are astonished (even angry) at China's efforts and take actions with ulterior motives.

The Trump administration announced it would suspend funding to the WHO, and the WHO criticized Washington for its failure to adopt a responsible attitude at an appropriate time. Japan is conceited while Europe is in a mess. It is at this period of time that China fills the vacuum left by the Trump administration. This is what has happened after the US first withdrew from Paris Climate Agreement (Elacuerdo delclima de París), then from the UNESCO and Iran Nuclear Deal. The acts of the US have created a circumstance that has enabled China to redefine its role in the world.

Because of what has happened, many people worry that China will become a model to replace the Western civilization. The pandemic has exposed the weaknesses of the Western countries in terms of politics, society, industry and technology. Robert Zoellick, former president of the World Bank, said to the effect that we will finally have to face our own shortcomings and we should not blame others. To some extent, the pandemic is foreshadowing. With respect to the responses to the COVID-19 pandemic, Asia is leading the race as Europe lags behind.

IV. Globalization may be changed because of this pandemic, but it will not perish

Calling for de-globalization is a way of "punishing" China indirectly. The same logic applies when they bring the supply chains from China back to the US. It is believed that some benefits would be derived from decoupling from China but not without paying a high price. The COVID-19 pandemic is undoubtedly harming globalization, and may possibly change its mechanism; however, it does not follow that globalization is dead. On the contrary, COVID-19 may accentuate the leadership of China in a new type of globalization that stays away from the supporters of "new liberalism."

The first reason for the imminent death of globalization is that there is nervous tension in the present globalization system. Prior to the outbreak of this pandemic, globalization had to meet the challenge of a mounting wave of populism driven by dissatisfaction with the economy in Europe, the US, Latin America and other regions. In addition, the pandemic occurred at a time when intercontinental strategic competition and trade war were intensified, which has eroded the basis of trust that supports globalization. It is in this sense that the COVID-19 pandemic has delivered the last blow to globalization.

There is always discontentment with globalization, although it has overcome many serious crises. The trend of globalization continues after going through two world wars, the Cold War, and the more recent anti-terrorism war. Globalization has also survived pandemic diseases such as the influenza pandemic (mistakenly called "Spanish influenza") in 1918, the Severe Acute Respiratory Syndrome (SARS) in 2003, the influenza A virus subtype H1N1 in 2009 and 2010 and the recent outbreak of Ebola.

The latest anti-globalization voice is not something new. Over the past decades, globalization has survived large-scale protests across the world. One of the setbacks that globalization meets is the withdrawal of the United Kingdom (UK) from the European Union (EU) that has been completed after a tortuous process of three and a half years when two prime ministers served their terms, displaying both the stability and vulnerability of the globalization system.

The second reason for the imminent death of globalization is more direct, which is about why coronavirus leads to the retrogression of globalization. According to this view, globalization is the chief culprit for the spread of the COVID-19 pandemic, or at least partly so. Some hold that the relatively rapid spread of coronavirus around the world can be attributed to the convenience brought about by international travel, but seen at a deeper level, it is resulted from globalization. In fact, blocking traffic and breaking the global connection have become the cornerstone of the international society in responding to the COVID-19 pandemic.

Virus is part of the nature. Epidemic diseases existed even before the initiation of today's globalization, and will probably remain so for a long time to come. Almost 20 years ago, airports began to conduct stringent security checks after the September 11 terrorist attack. Likewise, it can be imagined that all countries will reconsider their health control at the ports of entry.

Of course, corresponding measures should be taken with a long-term view. Out of health considerations, the US conducted health checks on immigrants entering the Ellis Island a century ago. As a response to the present the COVID-19 pandemic, tourists having travelled through Asia, the Middle East and some other regions are required to have their body temperature taken before they enter the territories of some countries. These measures merely represent an additional health test, and do not mean the end of international travel.

The third reason for the imminent death of globalization, and probably the most noteworthy one, is the fiasco of internationalism at the onset of this crisis. The countries throw blames to each other as to who should be held accountable for this crisis, killing the possibility of conducting major international cooperation. Changes occur with medical assistance even within the supranational entities like the EU. Each country concentrates on serving its own people; some countries even attempt to restrict the return of air flights.

These deficiencies are real and bound to bring changes. Following the rapid spread of COVID-19, each country takes more proactive measures to manage its own medical and health care industry to ensure that it maintains the capability of producing important supplies including face masks, respirators and prescribed medicines when it is confronted by an emergency. Many countries have adopted similar practical approaches to monitor the foundations of their national defense industry. Therefore, the changes that will occur in the medical and health care industry are not new practices, and they will not deliver a fatal blow to globalization.

Most importantly, globalization will go on because there is no change to its inner driving force, although there may be changes to its form. As what have happened for thousands of years, all countries need to continue to provide each other with commodities and services. Some countries are in need of a constant supply of natural resources, others will need inexpensive labor forces, and still others will be entitled to the opportunities to introduce foreign talents, skills and capitals. All countries need to trade with each other, as what they have done most of the time in history. The connections between different parts of the world that have been formed in the process of globalization over recent decades will not be broken easily, because many people have friends and family members who live abroad.

The outbreak of the COVID-19 pandemic will not affect the progress of telecommunication technologies by which information is transmitted to all parts of the world at an increasingly rapid speed. In fact, with the recent increase in telecommuting, the whole world is moving faster towards forging closer ties through online networks.

International cooperation will continue, because it is imperative to do so. If the whole world wants to defeat a disease that transcends national boundaries, all countries must work together to respond to the pandemic. Otherwise the virus may reappear in another place after it is beaten in one place, and nullify any victories achieved by any country alone.

V. Concluding Remarks

The crushing defeat suffered by the West at the onset of the COVID-19 pandemic aggravates the antagonism towards China, and is manifested as creating an atmosphere of being hostile to China. From the legal perspective, "demanding compensation" is a baseless request; yet it does not discourage the continued employment of unconventional stratagems for political, ideological and strategic reasons.

The COVID-19 pandemic has become a weapon of confrontation between the "China Model" and the "Model of Western Liberalism." As far as the present results are concerned, the China Model that is extolled by the WHO seems to have achieved success in the fight against the pandemic. China is extensively acclaimed for its success in this regard. The model established by China in responding to the pandemic has been modified before it is applied in many countries. Compared with some Western countries, China has saved more lives with its relatively successful control measures.

However, this does not mean that a system whereby more lives can be protected will become a universal choice. China believes that the selection of a political system by any country is to a large extent linked with the country's history and culture. Countries differ from each other in their culture and history. China has never tried to promote its political system worldwide, nor will it do so in the future, especially in case of emergency. Such a view is a component of the philosophy of China's diplomatic policies. Over decades, China has been exploring a path suited to its own national conditions, with the aim of realizing development and improving the people's quality of life.

The worries of Western countries reflect their rejection of China's political system. Some people still think that the model of liberalism is the best and universally applicable model, and that they have no reason to worry that other countries will draw from China's successful experience. It is this mentality that prevents these countries from drawing experience and lessons of China in its efforts to prevent and control the epidemic.

The world economy is moving towards the largest crisis ever since the Great Depression in 1929. The anxious warning given by the supporters of superpower demonstrates that the superpower may possibly lose its global position as a result of this pandemic crisis, and that this superpower is frantically looking for a "chief culprit." The COVID-19 pandemic confirms the efficacy of the governance approach of the East Asia in comparison with omission by the West. Such efficacy aggravates the anxiety of the US. Therefore, China is regarded by the US as a menacing threat because of its economic and technological development. However, if Donald Trump attempts to attack China to maintain the position of the US as a superpower, such attack will probably give rise to the situation that runs counter to what he wishes. The COVID-19 pandemic may accelerate the pace of China towards its leadership in the world.

Once Upon A Time in Hollywood – Objections to Slavoj Žižek

[Brazil] Cristiano Capovilla

Edited by Liu Xinxin[1]

About the Author

Cristiano Capovilla is a professor and philosopher at Federal University of Maranhã in Brazil. He has been teaching at various colleges and universities for more than 20 years. Cristiano Capovilla graduated from the Department of Philosophy, Federal University of Maranhã with a bachelor's degree, and graduated from Federal University of Piauí with a master's degree and PhD in philosophy. He also got a master's degree in science from State University of Rio de Janeiro. He is the director of the Maurício Grabois Foundation in the State of Maranhã.

---

1   Liu Xinxin, assistant research fellow of the Academy of Marxism, Chinese Academy of Social Sciences.

Abstract

The article on coronavirus by Slavoj Žižek is widely distributed overseas, and his vilification of Wuhan is not something new. Why the Western countries stigmatize China? And why the Western countries are ineffective in fighting the COVID-19 epidemic? It is necessary to find the reason within the system rather than discrediting China on the source of coronavirus.

I just read the text of "Popular Philosopher" Slavoj Žižek about the Coronavirus epidemic: "El coronavirus es um golpe al capitalismo a lo Kill Bill ...", included in a collection that recently published. Before anything, the book's cover catches the attention, with a design that suggests a colony of bats. By adding the image with the word *soup*, we retake one of the first fake news coming from the beginning of the pandemic. This misinformation, already duly denied by WHO,[1] shows how much eurocentrism is strong to qualify the unequal, the other. It is really terrifying that the suggestion of differences between civilized and barbarians be made even in the socioculture dimensions of feeding.

The unusual cover of the collection dialogs with the contents of the text of the Slovenian philosopher. From the beginning, Žižek does not hide his cheer about the debacle of Chinese communism from the pandemic onwards. He speculates that, like what happened in the former USSR, COVID-19 would be a kind of "Chernobyl nuclear factory" of the 21st century. It is exactly the same point federal deputy Eduardo Bolsonaro, son of President Bolsonaro, got used to state in order

---

1   According to the World Health Organization (WHO), there is no scientific evidence that "bat soup" was responsible for the spread of the new coronavirus in China. Source: https://saude.gov.br/fakenews/46240-sopa-de-morcego-e-o-coronavirus-e-fake-news?fbclid=IwAR1tnjZ7Am6w4pGJaQ2UWfLfNNgS1p0nFd1GTCFmqdPJhm2. Accessed on: April 15, 2020.

to attack China.[1] The finding that Žižek gets to is that China's fall will require from us "reinventing communism based on trust in people and science." (2020, p.22) The virus, such as in the film "Kill Bill 2," from the US director Quentin Tarantino, would have applied a kung-fu's mortal knock not only against China, but "against the global capitalist system." (2020, p.23) Following the Hollywood screenplay, we can stay in our quarantine waiting, talking and watching both fall dead after a certain time.

But where does this belief in the inevitable death of communist China and the capitalist system come from? It comes from the conviction that the "catastrophe" of the virus will lead humaniy to "rethink the basic characteristics of society." (2020, p.24) The natural "catastrophe" is exactly the exogenous cause that will lead to build "some efficient type of global coordination" (2020, p.25) opposite to the current political and economic system. A kind of rebellion caused by natural forces, of which the "drought, heat waves, massive torments" (2020, p.25) are also part of it.

Žižek supposes that the virus produced a contamination equality among the nations, classes and individuals: "We are all in the same boat," (2002, p.25) he sentences. This Phenomenon of the pandemic will be the mobile for an "urgent reorganization of the global economy" (2020, p.27) beyond the markets. It will be, therefore, through an external agent, the SARS-CoV-2 virus, that we will have, at last, an efficient cause to lead us to this new supportive system, a kind of communitarian UN, which will impose to the Nation-states the necessary adjustments to the social transformation of the new times. It will be an hybrid system between liberalism and communism, a conjunction between individual freedoms and the need for radical changes in global capitalism, he prophesied.

Far from Hollywood dreams and movies, the truth is that this equality of

---

1 "Eduardo Bolsonaro diz que culpa de pandemia do coronavírus é da China," March 18, 2020, see https://noticias.uol.com.br/politica/ultimas-noticias/2020/03/18/sem-provas-eduardo-bolsonaro-diz-que-culpa-da-pandemia-e-da-china.htm.

contamination is purely abstract, since in the objective reality it occurs within a framework of deep economic inequality between nations and social classes. In São Paulo the highest proportion of deaths does not respect age groups or comorbidities, but exclusively the victims' addresses, that is, more people die in the most excluded areas of the city, where sanitation problems, the lack of hospitals and the low income make residents more exposed to disease. New York data shows that black, latin and poor people are those who die of causes related to COVID-19.[1] Contamination, far from being a major equalizer of economic and social differences, exposes the deep deformations of our accumulation and lack system, revealing the eurocentric, classical and racist character of the egalitarian visions about the spread of the pandemic.

Now, as Žižek applies in his analyzes an external, unique and universal rule to assess the global pandemic, nothing more makes than obtain a distorted political, economic and social vision, hiding with the veil of ignorancy the heterogeneity among nations and, within these, asymmetries among social classes. It is clear that there is no natural law in the virus, a kind of intrinsic justice to the natural environment, which would come outside the social system to judge us, to punish us and, mainly, to be the redeemer of the illnesses bequested by our relations and ways of production of collective life.

If in capitalist system social relations become natural forces and the natural ones become living, so we should not also convert human conceptions such as equality and justice in natural forces, because they are political and social conditions. Therefore, they are submitted to history and not to physics or biology. There is no reason to exchange one metaphysics by another. None of them solves the problem.

With this formulation, I wonder: would Žižek be the heir of what in recent past

---

1   "Coronavírus mata negros e pobres de forma desproporcional nos EUA," Abr. 15, 2020, https://www1.folha.uol.com.br/mundo/2020/04/coronavirus-mata-negros-e-pobres-de-forma-desproporcional-nos-eua.shtml.

was called Western Marxism?

The Italian philosopher Domenico Losurdo answers this question in a scatching way: "the success that specially Žižek enjoys in our days leads us to think of not a recovery, but of a last breath of Western Marxism." (2018, p.167) This is because, since the Fall of the Berlin Wall and the disintegration of the USSR, this tradition of Western Left thought has disregarded in its diagnoses of international relations the analytical key of the fight against imperialism. The refusal of the role of colonialism and of anti-imperialist struggles led these thinkers to set up an abstract view of the capitalist power system.

Žižek, for example, divides the world between "authoritarian and non-authoritarian capitalism" (LUSURDO, 2018, p.167). He classifies, within the first group, countries such as China, Vietnam and Venezuela, and, in the second group, the rich Western nations like the USA, England and France, to mention only these countries. Within the "non-authoritarian" tradition are all the great colonialist metropolises of the past and imperialists of the present. But, while Democrat Lyndon B. Johnson was elected the 36th President of the United States in 1964, and enacted laws on civil rights and social security, at the same time, he ordered the huts of impotent and poor Vietnamese peasants be incinerated with napalm. All of that on behalf of imperialist geopolitics. What the Slovenian philosopher takes for "non-authoritarian" is only the "self-awareness of the dominant classes in Europe and in the USA" (LOSURDO, 2018, p.168), that is, the self-image they make of themselves as colonial metropolises. Under this perspective, he disregards the entire imperialist power system, neglecting the necessary anti-imperialist reaction of the invaded, looted and blocked peoples. This same discursive logic seems to be projected in the arguments about the current pandemic.

In my opinion the main question is: what transformations may suffer the State-nation in a society under the pandemic? This answer may only be given in the praxis of the political and institutional fight. The liberal State has shown itself fragile to face the challenge that threatens the nations. Without instruments of action, without planning and with markets in jamns, liberalism is put in check before national communities. Such shortcomings are highlighted in contrast to Chinese communism and its "Project Based Planning." From the end of February, when the Slovenian philosopher wrote the article, to the half of April, when I am answering, China has passed from the main victim of an exogenous natural disease to the most important social and political protagonist in the fight against the new virus. Exactly because he did not consider it, the prognosis of Žižek on China did not resist two months, evidencing that it was more a subjective desire from the author than properly a serious and compromised with reality reflection.

The US, precisely the heroes of Hollywood films, those who used to save the world of "natural disasters," are the ones who most suffer the effects of the pandemic, not only by action of the virus itself, but by mistaken political and ideological decisions. The US drama exposes to the world that the *american way of life* is the jungle law, where only the strongest ones survive. Maybe it would better for Žižek, when referring to the coronavirus pandemic, to rescue another Tarantino film: "Once upon a time in Hollywood."

Unlike what says Žižek, virus made the Chinese State-nation respond in an unprecedent and amazing way to this new threat. It made and is making the difference in the victory of society against the natural fear, presenting itself in conditions to propose an offensive act. What the World should question itself is why USA and Europe are being defeated in the battle against COVID-19 and China, a really communist country, is going to beat it? Perhaps the answer is inside, not outside of the historical-social relationships.

References:

LOSURDO, Domenico. *O marxismo ocidental: como nasceu, como morreu, como pode renascer*. Tradução Ana Maria Chiarini e Diego Silveira Coelho Ferreira. São Paulo: Boitempo, 2018.

Žižek, Slavoj. El Coronavirus es um golpe al capitalismo a lo Kill Bill ... (27 de Febrero). In: *Sopa de Wuhan. Pensamiento contemporaneo em tiempos de pandemias*. Pablo Amadeo (Org.) La Plata: Editorial ASPO (Aislamiento Social Preventivo y Obligatorio), 2020.

The Fight Against COVID-19 – an Interview with Victor Wallis

[America] Victor Wallis

Edited by Zhuo Mingliang[1]

About the Author

Dr. Victor Wallis graduated from the Department of Politics of Columbia University in 1970, and taught at the Department of Political Science at St. Lawrence University and the Department of Political Science at Indiana University-Purdue University at Indianapolis. He is a professor at the Department of Political Science in Berklee College of Music in the US.

Wallis has a lot of books to his credit during his teaching career of nearly half a century. He mainly specializes in ecology and technology, American society and politics, and Latin American politics. His publications in recent years include: *Socialist Practice: Histories and Theories* (2020), *Democracy Denied: Five Lectures on U.S. Politics* (2019), *Red-Green Revolution: The Politics and Technology of Ecosocialism* (2018) and others. He is a long-term contributor to *Monthly Review*, an American left-wing magazine, and serves as the managing editor of *Socialism and Democracy*.

---

1   Zhuo Mingliang, contributing researcher of the World Socialism Research Center, Chinese Academy of Social Sciences, and visiting professor of Nanchang Institute of Technology.

Abstract

The pandemic has triggered an economic depression of calamitous proportions around the world. What the American government does for responding to the spread of the epidemic are far from being desired. Moreover, Trump shamelessly engaged in activities that abused his power for personal gains. In contrast, the responses made by socialist countries like China and Cuba to major emergencies reflect the mix between executive decrees on the one hand and popular initiative and participation on the other. The quality of universal services would be more dependably assured within a fully socialist framework.

I. The US government falls short in response to the COVID-19 epidemic

The spread of the virus to other countries began already before late March. As for why the initial spread was so rapid, it is well known that COVID-19 is exceptionally contagious and that those who are infected by it do not necessarily show symptoms. These two traits, in combination, guarantee rapid spread unless certain requirements have been met.

Most directly, there must be ample supplies of the appropriate diagnostic tests, personal protective gear (masks, gloves, hand sanitizers, etc., especially for healthcare workers), and ventilators.

At a more basic level, there must be an adequate healthcare infrastructure. This means that there must be enough hospitals and enough healthcare professionals and support staff to be able to respond effectively to emergencies. It also means that all persons must be able to get diagnosed and treated free of charge.

A further requirement is that policy decisions should be informed by scientific opinion, and not based on business prospects or on jockeying for political advantage. Expert knowledge should be widely diffused so that everyone can understand the need for whatever measures are taken.

At a broader institutional level, there are certain additional requirements. There should be universal "sick leave," and there should be unemployment compensation for all those whose jobs are terminated. Further, no person should lack housing (without which self-quarantining is impossible). Also, no distinction should be made, in matters of healthcare, between citizens or legal residents and those lacking such status (given that any inhabitant of the society is a potential transmitter of the virus). Finally, the government must have both the capacity and the political will to order the emergency mobilization of resources as needed, for everything from educating the public to assuring food supplies to rapidly building temporary hospitals.

In all these critical dimensions, the United States falls short. But on top of these shortcomings, which are not new, the present administration has reacted to the crisis in a uniquely perverse manner. For weeks, even after being informed of the pandemic, it scoffed at the danger and refused to adopt a diagnostic test that had been made available by the World Health Organization. Instead of promoting internal and international solidarity, it encouraged scapegoating by ethnicity, intensified its already devastating sanctions against Iran and Venezuela, and tried to obstruct Cuba's remarkable program of international medical aid.

As if all this were not enough, the president engages in the most shameless forms of corrupt self-serving. At his daily news conferences, he either excludes critical questions or denounces those who raise them. He requires that his name be printed on all relief-checks. His apportionment of federal aid to the various states is determined not by their respective needs but rather by whether he likes or dislikes their governors. In defiance of medical opinion, he promotes a drug of uncertain merit in whose production a former lawyer of his has a financial interest.

I don't deny the dangers of a prolonged shutdown, which has its own damaging effects on public health.

II. The clash between capitalist principles and human need

The capitalist approach to healthcare is epitomized by the deficiencies of the US system. The essence of this approach is to treat healthcare as a commodity and to make treatment dependent upon a person's ability to pay. Of course, this may be partially mediated by insurance, but if the insurance is also capitalist, then the individual may still be at risk of heavy financial burden if not the actual denial of necessary medical procedures (even with the COVID-19 emergency, diagnostic testing is frequently denied to persons lacking insurance). The absurdity of such an arrangement, if not apparent earlier, has been highlighted by the current crisis, in which millions of workers suddenly lost their health insurance along with their jobs.

The clash between capitalist principles and human need is especially striking in the sphere of healthcare because we find here an extraordinarily glaring discrepancy between the potential cost of a recommended medical procedure and the capacity of a person of average or low income to pay for it. The notion of measuring need through the market fails here so completely that even in otherwise capitalist countries, it has been widely recognized that the provision of healthcare must be informed by socialist principles. Still, the actual implementation of such an approach depends on pressure from the organized working class (which, as a political force, has been notoriously weak in the United States). And there remains the problem that a capitalist regime will tend to weaken public health guarantees as it has, for example, in England, whose National Health Service is increasingly undercut by privatizing measures.[1]

A more thoroughgoing socialist approach presupposes the socialist reorganization of society, which makes possible a preventive approach to healthcare. Moreover, if a socialist approach is applied not just to insurance but to the health

---

1   John Pilger, "The Dirty War on the NHS" (December 2019 interview), see https://www.youtube.com/watch?v=rHZcXrc9_wk.

services themselves, then it becomes easier to allocate skills and supplies on the basis of need.

A socialist approach to healthcare thus goes beyond responding just to market demand or to private interests and instead builds an infrastructure that can respond to emergency needs. This was strikingly shown in China.

The capitalist framework, by contrast, not only suffers from the drawbacks I have noted; in addition, in its current "neoliberal" form, it has increasingly prioritized cost-cutting. In the same way that manufacturing industry, using new technologies, turns more and more to "just in time" production (not building up inventories, thereby risking sudden shortages), so also the healthcare industry, in its drive for "efficiency," closes down hospitals and reduces its total numbers of beds, which then come up short in the event of an emergency.

The US system uniquely embodies capitalist priorities not only in its minimizing of any "public interest" restraint, but also in its obsession with being the world's top military power. Where socialism encourages its adherents to view the international realm as a sphere of cooperation, capitalism highlights competition and domination. The US government thus explicitly defined its global role (in the National Security Strategy document of 2002) as requiring unchallenged military supremacy. This means that there can never be, in its eyes, any limit to "defense" expenditures, but that – in consequence of this – all other budget items are under severe constraint. The military emphasis is supposedly justified on grounds of "national security." And yet what can more severely undermine a country's security than the government's inability to protect its population against a deadly pandemic?

III. The COVID-19 epidemic has cast an unprecedented spotlight on the fundamental flaws of capitalist society

The pandemic has triggered an economic depression of calamitous proportions. As of this moment (late April 2020), more than 26 million US jobs have been lost since its onset, with total unemployment projected to reach 30% of the labor force. The world configuration will surely be affected by the relative speed with which various countries can return to normal levels of economic activity. The US is at a disadvantage in this respect.

Beyond this, the pandemic has cast an unprecedented spotlight on the fundamental flaws of capitalist society. It has underscored the incapacity of the world's most powerful capitalist government to respond to urgent human need. Corporations as well as key agencies of government prioritize profits and accumulation over public health. In the words of a huge sign recently displayed by a group of New York workers, "Capitalism is the virus."

Capitalism not only enables the spread of COVID-19; it will also use public health concerns as a pretext for augmenting its longstanding surveillance and disruption of dissident political activity. Its resort to such measures will increase as the economic hardship resulting from the depression brings a rise in mass discontent. Even before the onset of COVID-19, popular majorities in the US supported the idea of universal free healthcare. In the near term, however, it is clear that the ruling class's opposition to this idea will prevail. The US government, already seen as an aggressive force on the world stage, will then also come to be perceived as both ineffective and undemocratic at home.

Some US politicians have blamed China for failing to contain COVID-19 and for spreading it to the world, making it a costly global pandemic. This type of claim by US politicians is an attempt to divert attention from their own failure to provide the necessary leadership in overcoming the pandemic. The more severe the economic and public health situation becomes, the more important it will be for them to blame the people's sufferings on some external agent. In the present case, where the pandemic has triggered an economic collapse, the systemic failure is more glaring than ever. Blaming China is an attempt not only to shift the focus of popular anger, but also to discredit any impulse to cite China's response to the crisis as a positive model.

IV. Socialism is more effective in dealing with momentous public emergency events

What I have said regarding the response to pandemics applies to any public emergency event. In all such cases, routine activities and responsibilities are disrupted. The capitalism-fostered illusion of individual self-sufficiency collapses completely. Any possible rescue depends on a whole community. While the corresponding sense of solidarity was the norm in earlier epochs and did not disappear completely under capitalism, it maintained only a marginal existence, often overwhelmed by an aggressive ideology of rugged individualism. The resulting "war of all against all" mentality now leads a growing sector of the US population to respond to the pandemic by arming itself, causing a sudden sharp increase in the sale of guns and bullets.

Solidarity still exists within families, among friends, and in voluntary associations (whether religious, cultural, or political), but there is no sense of solidarity at the level of US society as a whole. Exhortations to national unity remain purely ritualistic. The ubiquitous Trump slogan, "Make America great again," is widely and accurately understood to signify "Make America white again," as the remembered prosperity to which it harks back – in the post-1945 years of US global economic supremacy – largely excluded African Americans.

With the relative economic decline of the US since the mid-1970s, the working class suffered as a result of (1) the shift of manufacturing jobs to low-wage countries and (2) neoliberal policies imposed by both Democrats and Republicans. Trump's racist and xenophobic rhetoric draws attention away from these policies and encourages the white working class instead to view its misfortunes as being caused by immigrants, Muslims, and people of color.

Other recent disasters in the US illustrate further how, under unrestrained capitalism, private agendas of various kinds – often fueled by racism – can get in the way of attending to the common good. Another example arose during the vast

California forest fires of 2018. While the State augmented its firefighting crews by hiring prisoners at slave wages, private firefighting companies offered their rich customers a more rapid response on an exclusive basis.

It can be generally argued, for any public service, including healthcare and education as well as disaster-relief, that resources sucked into the private sector are in effect being drawn out of the public sector. When the entire population is served by the institutions in question (hospitals, schools, post offices, buses and subways, fire departments, etc.), then the services that they provide will be of higher quality than they would be if offered only to that portion of the public – the large majority – which cannot directly pay for them. This is because when the institutions in question are geared toward the entire population (in the context of a class-divided society), their operations are more likely to be properly supported by the government than if they were serving "only" the working class and middle class.

The approach of serving and being accountable to everyone is that of socialism. My immediate point is that the merits of this approach have long been evident even within an otherwise capitalist framework. The democratic dimension is implicitly socialistic, in that its achievements have depended on the initiative and support of the organized working class, and have had to face continuous capitalist-driven challenges, in the form of privatizations and budget cutbacks. The quality of universal services would be more dependably assured within a fully socialist framework.

This said, socialist responses may themselves take a variety of forms. The core question is that of the mix between executive decrees on the one hand and popular initiative and participation on the other. Executive decrees may show quicker results than the democratic approach, but they encourage a concentration of power that could have the effect of not only alienating people from performing their immediate tasks, but also undermining the long-range goal of building a classless society.

The fight against the epidemic is in part also a fight against the economic crash it has precipitated. The present moment is one in which there is at least, thanks to the epidemic as well as the depression, an enormous focusing of public attention on issues of common concern. As the situation is one of evident systemic failure, there should be more openness than usual to the consideration of radical alternatives.

The only possible basis for a long-term response to such pandemics is one that takes into account the underlying social and environmental conditions under which they arise. These include (thinking beyond the case of COVID-19): (1) geopolitical agendas that promote biological warfare research;[1] (2) corporate capitalist projects for the mass marketing of supposedly definitive vaccines against the next plague;[2] and (3) underlying all else, the wholesale destruction of natural habitats that has disrupted species-life, leading to the dispersion of viruses in unprecedented directions.

The environmental crisis itself has reached an acute phase. It does not manifest itself with the same intensity everywhere at once. But a pandemic, like massive floods or drought-induced forest fires, is one of a number of alarm signals that periodically crash into mass complacency, commanding everyone to pay heed to the more total disaster that threatens. To "win the fight against the epidemic" will require making it part of the broader struggle to reverse, so far as possible, the global assault on the natural environment. This struggle is obviously of concern to all people throughout the world, although, like the fight against COVID-19, it requires a clear understanding of the class interests that must be overcome.

---

1   For thorough discussion, see https://www.salon.com/2020/04/24/did-this-virus-come-from-a-lab-maybe-not--but-it-exposes-the-threat-of-a-biowarfare-arms-race/.
2   See the April 2015 Ted Talk by multi-billionaire entrepreneur Bill Gates, https://www.youtube.com/watch?v=6Af6b_wyi

The Community with Shared Future for Mankind as a Way out of the Global Emergency Caused by the COVID-19

[Spain] José Luis Centella Gómez

Edited by Zhu Weiwei[1]

About the Author

José Luis Centella Gómez was born on July 31, 1958. He is a politician, a member and former general secretary of the Central Committee of the Communist Party of Spain. On April 8, 2018, he was elected chairman of the Communist Party of Spain at the last session of its 20th Congress.

Abstract

The COVID-19 pandemic highlights all weaknesses of the capitalist system that puts economic interest first. The "Neo-liberalism" and the capitalist system already showed signs of decline prior to the outbreak of the pandemic, and this trend will be inevitably aggravated following the end of the crisis. The COVID-19 pandemic poses a challenge to all humanity. To address this crisis, the present global governance model should give way to a new global governance model that is based on multilateralism and the horizontal relations

---

1   Zhu Weiwei, associate research fellow of the Institute of Information, Chinese Academy of Social Sciences.

between countries. It is of important significance to develop the community of common destiny in this new global governance model. Through developing the community of common destiny, we will not only rid ourselves of the present emergency as soon as possible through mutual collaboration and resource sharing, but will also avoid running into similar crisis in the future, and contribute a comprehensive and sustainable concept of security that can be shared for the benefit of all human beings.

It is said that the COVID-19 epidemic is the most prominent systemic risk test in the field of public health that the world has faced since the World War II, highlighting the advantages and disadvantages of the governance capabilities of capitalist and socialist systems. Regarding to this topic, Centella Gómez Shared his opinion with us in the interview April 2020.

This crisis has revealed all the weaknesses of a capitalist system that subordinates life to economic interest. In this way, in Europe and the US there has not been a complete closure of activity because capitalist companies rule in governments and do not want to lose their benefits.

This circumstance has caused a higher rate of contagion because total confinement of the population has not been produced, since the capitalist market has imposed itself on medical health experts.

At the same time, the lack of market control leads to speculation on the value of medical and sanitary materials, so that tests to detect the disease could be done quickly by anyone with money, while most of the people have had to pass the Pandemic without being able to do these screening tests.

The Pandemic has not provoked a new framework of international relations, but if it is to accelerate the processes of change, in this sense, it is important to bear in mind that the decline of the so-called Neoliberal Globalization, of lacking capitalism, predates the crisis caused by COVID-19, because it was increasingly evident that the problems of humanity cannot be solved with a system of international relations based on a unipolar world, in which the profits of the great powers are obtained at the cost of the losses of the least developed States , in what is called zero sum theory.

What has happened is that the pandemic crisis is making this decline worse, causing a new danger, because if this neoliberal globalization was negative for humanity, the alternative that some capitalist thinkers of closing borders may be even worse with all these obstacles to international trade, and the aggravation of the unilateral nature of international relations.

Therefore it is evident that the exit from the crisis caused by the Pandemic will have consequences for the future of the Planet, the question is that these changes may be positive to improve the life conditions of the humanity.

It is a reality that at the beginning of the crisis some believed that this crisis seemed to affect only China and it could mean the decline of the Chinese-style socialism system, achieving the re-position of the capitalist West as the center of world power.

However, the way in which China faced, controlled and defeated the Pandemic as well as the solidarity that China is showing towards the rest of the Planet, while the Great Capitalist States were overwhelmed by the growth of the Pandemic, has led to a Increased sympathy of many western people who had reluctance towards China and now begin to value the Chinese system very positively, so this question means that we have a better future perspective for Socialism after the medical health crisis.

Severe infectious diseases are the enemies of all mankind. In my opinion, this emergency situation that the entire planet is experiencing makes it necessary to give way to a new World Governance based on multilateralism and horizontal relations in the States, which develops fair trade of mutual benefit in which everyone wins, burying The theory of zero sum, making great changes in the international order, and also in the international institutions.

In this approach to this new World Governance, the proposal made by the President of the People's Republic of China, Xi Jinping, to build a community with a shared future for mankind, which adds volunteers and efforts to make sense of the rest of the planet. An opportunity, first of all to overcome the Pandemic and then to develop a new world order from a cooperation between the different States that can achieve common objectives for all the inhabitants of the Planet until they are able to have the right to a dignified life, while adding efforts to fight together in the future emergency situations as the one is experiencing humanity right now.

Building a community with a shared future for *humanity* is what it can allow, not only to facilitate a faster exit from the current emergency situation through mutual cooperation and the possibilities of sharing resources, but it can help us to avoid situations like the current one would be repeated again, developing a comprehensive and sustainable shared security concept for the benefit of the whole Humanity.

No one can deny that in the current world there is total interdependence between all countries and territories, the question is to be able to face this interrelation from reciprocal cooperation that manages to share resources and technical advances to multiply the profit in a shared way, developing clear rules that help and protect the weakest and most vulnerable States from the aggressions of the most powerful and developed States.

To begin with, an emergency crisis like the one humanity is experiencing in these times shows us that the crisis does not respect borders or continents; it makes international cooperation necessary, promoting the role of the United Nations in order to recover the application of the values and principles included in the UN Charter, because there can be no World Governance without an Institution that represents the democratic and representative character and that has control over international economic institutions, to make them more useful to the countries that will suffer the most. In an emergency situation, in this sense, international economic cooperation must undergo great changes to establish rules that affect better use of the economy to improve the quality of life of those affected by the consequences of the crisis.

In these times, the development of the productive forces, the technological advances, the medical discoveries allow at the moment to face emergency situations like the current one, it is only necessary to end a neoliberal market that has neither control nor moral to develop rules and controls that promote the relationship between the use of medical techniques together with the economic policies that are proposed to overcome the crisis, which has to be focused on the general interest, always under the direction of the State as a reference for the defense of the Common Good.

This is the basic question, manage to get humanity out of this solidary crisis, convinced that only the joint work of all peoples can guarantee a future life for humanity.

Four Reasons for China to Secure Victory Against the COVID-19 Epidemic

[Germany] Frank Schumann

Edited by Lei Xiaohuan[1]

About the Author

Frank Schumann is the president of Edition Ost Berlin, a well-known publishing house in Germany, and the former editor-in-chief of *Daily Newspaper (Tageszeitung)* in East Germany. He was born in the German Democratic Republic (GDR) in 1951. He served in the People's Navy of the GDR from 1970 to 1973 when he joined the Socialist Unity Party of Germany. From 1978 to 1991, Schumann worked at *Junge Welt*, where he served as the director of its Science/Publicity Department, chief editor of its culture section and its editor-in-chief. *Junge Welt* was the newspaper with the largest circulation (1.6 million copies) in the GDR.

Following the reunification of Germany in October, 1990, he established Edition Ost Berlin in 1991, and becomes a publisher and political commentator. He had compiled and published the books by politicians including former general secretaries of the Socialist Unity Party of Germany such as Walter Ulbricht, Erich Honecker and Egon Krenz, and Hans Modrow, former prime minister of the GDR, and Gregor Gysi and Sahra Wagenknecht, leaders of The Left, a political party in Germany.

---

1   Lei Xiaohuan, assistant research fellow of the Academy of Marxism, Chinese Academy of Social Sciences.

Abstract

To Marxists, the COVID-19 pandemic is not simply a medical issue. We need to do an in-depth study and analysis from the political perspective. The COVID-19 epidemic does not change the ownership of the means of production in capitalist countries, and the class question still exists. Therefore, the judgment of the capitalist countries on the measures adopted by China in fighting COVID-19 epidemic can be categorized as a class question. We must be keenly aware that no matter how Western countries slander China, China has been a success in its fight against the COVID-19 epidemic, and such a success is closely linked with China's socialist system.

At present, about the COVID-19 pandemic we have at least four problems. The first is the medical problem, the second is the economic impact of the pandemic. The third problem area is the social element. And fourthly, it is about politics and how to deal with these three problems.

The fourth problem is of course the key question for Marxists. All other issues – economy, society and medicine – are subordinated in that they are dictated by the politics of the ruling class. The conditions of production determine the character of a society – and thus also the policy in dealing with the corona virus.

The virus overcomes state borders, but not social borders. Because although the virus affects all areas and changes a lot, it does not change the character of the production situation. Ownership of the means of production remains, and so does the private appropriation of the jointly generated added value.

So the class question continues. Everything else derives from this. Also the judgment of the West, i.e. the capitalist states, about the measures taken by the socialist People's Republic of China in the fight against the Corona virus is class question. The measures taken by the party are "undemocratic" and "violate human rights," it said. These allegations ceased when – firstly – the so-called democratic states resorted to the same restrictive regulations because – secondly – the measures in China had proven successful. Which of course was denied. The official figures released by China, the media spread, are certainly "beautified," "styled," "fake." In addition, it could not be admitted that the western states had taken the same measures in the fight against the corona virus that the maligned People's Republic of China had taken as an example. Only the World Health Organization (WHO) said that, for which it was sharply criticized.

No matter what China did or failed to do, it was basically communist propaganda. "Communists are naturally lying." It wasn't said so clearly, but the media suggested it. And still suggest it. The arguments are cheap and often wrong.

In this context, the *Neue Zürcher Zeitung* mentioned that Beijing has "filled a vacuum" in the UN system for years, "that has arisen from Washington's demonstrative lack of interest in multilateral forums." The "demonstrative lack of interest" is a friendly description of the hegemonic interest of the United States in dictatorial stamping on the world. The United States cannot cope with a multipolar world. "America First" is basically the derivation of the first of The ten Commandments into the language of politics. It reads: "I am the Lord, your God, you should not have other gods besides me." That means: Those who do not submit to the will of the United States must face sanctions.

After the numbers of sick and deceased in China had already decreased, those in the USA continued to increase dramatically. In mid-April, the United States took the top spot in both infections and deaths, leaving Western Europe behind.

These were facts that could not be eliminated with anti-communist, anti-Chinese propaganda. And even if the topic is mainly treated as a medical and psycho-mental one in the media, the actual topic increasingly shimmers through. The core of capitalism is capital, and if nothing can be earned anymore because the economy is paralyzed and therefore no profit is produced, then capital becomes restless and shows concern. At the beginning of April, the most important German news magazine showed a bundle of banknotes on the title that was visibly eroded.

"The bankruptcy virus" stood above it. "How Corona infects our economy, eats jobs and prosperity." (*Der Spiegel*, April 4, 2020) At the same time, a major Berlin daily newspaper headlined "Pandemic threatens billions of jobs" (*Der Tagesspiegel*, April 8, 2020). That wasn't wrong, but it was only half the truth. And half truths are sometimes whole lies. The whole truth is that workers lose their jobs – employers lose their earnings and shareholders lose their returns.

With social demagogy, the bourgeois press turned the fundamental problem of capitalist production into a problem for workers. So the press didn't ask the system question. She didn't even ask: Why did China manage to get the virus under control while we are trying to alleviate the symptoms with a lot of money?

The Chancellor and the Federal President fled to the front by addressing the German people with TV speeches. Usually, the head of government and head of state speak out only once a year – for Christmas and New Year. The ratings of the speeches were unusually high, so many viewers did not even have football matches of the national team or Bayern Munich. The two top politicians calmed the state people and spread confidence. The Federal President even claimed: "We are now at a crossroads."

Of course, he did not mean the decision for this or another social system, but for individual behavior. "Either everyone for themselves, elbows out," or "remains the newly awakened commitment for the other, for society?" And translated globally: "Are we looking for a way out in the world, or are we falling back into isolation and going it alone?" The head of state summoned solidarity internally and externally. "We will be a different society after this crisis. We don't want to be a fearful, no suspicious society. But we can be a society with more trust, with more respect and with more respect and with more confidence."

The physicist at the Federal Chancellery became a little more specific: "Don't believe rumors, just the official communications, which we always have translated into many languages. We are a democracy. We do not live from coercion, but from shared knowledge and participation. "In other words, where there is no democracy (i.e. what is meant by democracy in the West), there is compulsion and ignorance.

Soberly, one has to state that the German leadership remains unchanged on its old path. The "pathway" was only rhetorical.

It must be stated with the same sobriety that the Chinese were successful in the fight against the virus because, firstly, they were able to concentrate all their strength. Secondly, because they were not, like the leaders of the western world, arrogant to master everything, to know everything, to be able to do everything. The arrogance of the alleged superiority is obviously alien to the leaders of China. And thirdly, they managed to motivate the people and convince them that the measures taken were correct and necessary. Without the discipline and unity of the whole people, the fight against COVID-19 would not have been successful. All of this was causally related to the character of society, which is socialist. Just as the socialist Soviet Union in the Great Patriotic War between 1941 and 1945 was able to join forces against the fascist enemy and defeat it, China also succeeded in mobilizing all social forces.

It does not seem to matter that you might hesitate at first to avoid panic. That one was careful with information and did not immediately alarm the world public. It was important to act with determination. And with the other countries solidary help and support has been and will be provided. The People's Republic of China has acted in an exemplary manner and has thus gained a reputation in the world.

The demagogy with which the current pandemic is treated in the western media and by western politicians has a forerunner: the Spanish flu of 1918. At that time, it was believed that between 50 and 100 million human lives were claimed worldwide. So considerably more deaths than the whole world war cost in 1914-1918.

The Spanish flu, an influenza pandemic, did not come from Spain. Most scientists today assume that it originated in the United States and came to Europe with the soldiers. Spain was a neutral country at the time, the press also reported openly about the flu illness of the Spanish king, which is why the term "Spanish flu" became common abroad. Because in the censored newspapers of the belligerent states the illnesses were not reported. At most as the supposed weapon of war of the opponent. The Americans claimed that the flu was smuggled into the United States from canned fish poisoned by the Germans.

Again, why was the People's Republic of China's fight against COVID-19 successful? Because humanism is an essential element of a socialist society. The human being with his needs is at the center of all social efforts – not the interests of a certain group, not that of a minority or an organization. And the character of socialist society also allows for long-term goals and goals. This is not only visible in the strategy of "two hundred years." This is also evident in health policy. At the National Conference on Hygiene and Health in summer 2016, Xi Jinping referred to the "long-term efforts" to raise health levels. "In promoting a healthy China, we should follow the chinese health development path and tackle major problems." This was clearly evident in the Corona crisis. Although in 2016 no one, including Xi Jinping, could have guessed what would emerge as a "serious problem" in Wuhan years later.

The Social and Economic Challenges that COVID-19 Presents to Humankind

[Brazil] Agnaldo dos Santos

Edited by Liu Xinxin[1]

About the Author

Agnaldo dos Santos PhD in Sociology. Assistant Professor of Political Economy at São Paulo State University (UNESP), Faculty of Philosophy and Sciences, Department of Political and Economic Sciences.

Abstract

The spread of coronavirus poses a huge challenge to humankind, and triggers worldwide debates on the future of the capitalist economy. Many countries and regions adopt fiscal austerity policies. The withdrawal of the UK from the EU, the election of Donald Trump as president of the US and the election of Jair Bolsonaro as president of Brazil all illustrate the changes to the political concepts in the present world. The COVID-19 epidemic is a test of the health system of all countries. Given the high probability that the fight against the epidemic will be a protracted one, economic reconstruction will

1 Liu Xinxin, assistant research fellow of the Academy of Marxism, Chinese Academy of Social Sciences.

become an issue of primary importance when people are faced with double challenges of the COVID-19 epidemic and the economic depression at the end of 2019. The economic reconstruction requires global solidarity to jointly overcome adversities. The more the problems with capitalist market economy are exposed, the more it is necessary to seek a new path. As the outbreak of COVID-19 exerts huge impacts upon the economy, people discuss whether there exist alternative development plans that are more inclusive. We will adopt a wait-and-see attitude toward how the progressive and leftist political forces will address this problem and how the socialist construction will meet the imminent challenges.

From the perspective of the biological sciences, it is not strange that epidemics generated by the transmission of bacteria and viruses accompany humanity throughout history. Some, such as the so-called "Black Plague" in medieval Europe (also in 14th-century Asia of the Common Era), and that mistakenly called "Spanish Flu," in the beginning of the 20th, left deep marks in the popular imagination and many reports in historical records. The pandemic situation generated by the spread of the COVID-19 coronavirus is especially tragic due to the rapid spread, the unique characteristics of this virus and its impact on the economy and health systems worldwide.

Since the World Health Organization (WHO) considered it, the spread of COVID-19 has sparked, in addition to the indispensable increase in health care, a worldwide debate on the future of the capitalist economy. Moreover, humanity itself, in the face of this enormous challenge. Can the capitalist market economy, and the widespread belief in the West of its "self-regulation," survive with the drastic reduction in production, circulation and services? Could the necessary state intervention in national economies, to encourage aggregate demand, mark the end of the neoliberal narrative? Will international solidarity increase, in the search for a treatment of the viral scourge, or will we enter a new "feudal era," with insulation of national economies and increased animosities and xenophobic nationalism?

What we can do now is to try to prospect for possible scenarios. What seems certain, however, is that we will not return to the scenario immediately before the start of the pandemic. Understanding the possibilities can create conditions for progressive forces around the world to seek to strive for a better world than today.

We will present in this small text, in an essay form, the general conditions in which the world found itself when the pandemic broke out, the ways in which different countries are currently trying to face the disease and the trends we can envision, from the perspective of the Global South (countries like Brazil, for example). We believe it is possible that the crisis generated by the pandemic will create conditions for greater international collaboration, but this is not certain and will not happen automatically.

I. The world before the new coronavirus pandemic

There is a consensus among political analysts that the claim for a unipolar world with the United States ahead, at the beginning of the 21st century, was seriously shaken. More particularly, after the 2008 Wall Street financial crisis. Since the end of the Cold War, with the disintegration of the Soviet Union, the world economy has accelerated its integration process, baptized by American analysts as "globalization."

The economic and political revenues prescribed by multilateral agencies under the influence of the United States, such as the International Monetary Fund (IMF) and the World Bank (WB), were for the economic integration of global value chains, forcing the specialization of economies. Many countries of recent industrialization have been forced to revert their characteristics to mere producers of *commodities* and consumers of imported manufactured goods. Moreover, the conservative political forces in these countries, line with this view, adopted fiscal austerity policies, indiscriminate privatization of strategic state enterprises, budget cuts in social services, deregulation of economic sectors, reduction of the number of civil servants etc..

Despite some financial crises throughout the 1990s and early 2000s, globalization oriented by the USA, Europe and Japan seemed irresistible. It is true that some countries of recent intensive industrialization, such as the People's Republic of China, or which have rebuilt themselves after deep crises, such as post-Boris Yeltsin Russia, have already emerged as important *players* on the global stage. However, the neoliberal hegemony of globalization seemed unchallenged.

Then came the global crisis of 2008, generated by the financial activities of *subprime loans*, which brought down stock exchanges around the world. Economic practice unequivocally contradicted the precepts of self-regulated markets, preached by neoliberal revenue. Nation states have been called upon to bail out large banks and companies to prevent even greater economic damage.

Despite the evidence, many political actors, both in the center and on the periphery of the geopolitical and economic system, have again defended the resumption of fiscal austerity plans. One of the consequences of the insistence of this agenda, which was totally or partially accepted by leftist parties, was the emergence of xenophobic and neo-fascist inspired speeches, as an easy way to combat unemployment and low economic growth. The electoral results that led to the withdrawal of the United Kingdom from the European Union ("Brexit") and the victories of Donald Trump in the United States and Jair Bolsonaro in Brazil, just to stay in these examples, show the new political state of mind around the world.

Increasing animosities between Trump's U.S. and the rising economies like China have taken on more dramatic tones in the current climate. Before the outbreak of the coronavirus pandemic, Trump already made clear his intention to open a trade war with China and other countries that are not completely aligned with his guidelines. This strategy was already expected, due to its campaign for re-election in 2020, but it became even more aggressive after the arrival of COVID-19 in American territory.

In fact, American hegemony showed signs of weakening, which were evidenced by the beginning of the pandemic. The postwar USA did not accept a basket of currencies suggested in Bretton Woods and imposed its dollar as an international means of payment. After 1973, it sets aside convertibility for gold, seeking to maintain its currency with its previous status. Not only because it can issue dollars, according to its needs, has it also used the currency as a form of economic pressure against non-aligned nation states.

The United States and its European partners systematically veto reform proposals in multilateral organizations, such as the United Nations, the World Bank and the International Monetary Fund. The growing importance of the G-20, a group of countries that includes, for example, China, Russia, Brazil, India and South Africa, has led to the elaboration of alternatives to the unilateral positions of the USA. The emergence of the BRICS, with the countries mentioned above, and the creation of the New Development Bank (NDB), despite proposing greater economic integration, is seen as a threat to US interests.

The controversial way in which former Brazilian President Dilma Rousseff was dismissed in 2016 and the subsequent victory of the extreme right with Jair Bolsonaro, Trump's rapprochement with Indian nationalists and the American president's permanent tension against Chinese and Russians must be understood in this perspective. Efforts to return to the *status quo ante*. The discursive violence with which the US presidency accuses China and the World Health Organization, on alleged responsibilities regarding the spread of the coronavirus pandemic across the planet, must be understood in this logic.

It is important to observe, then, the behavior of the different countries that face the severity of the pandemic, as it can give us clues about the possibilities that open up for cooperation or for increasing international tensions.

II. The battle against COVID-19 around the world

There are still doubts about how COVID-19 emerged. Despite the scientific importance of identifying the location of the appearance of this viral strain, the most important thing now is to build the best ways to face the pandemic, especially in the treatment of those who have been infected.

A characteristic of the disease, widely publicized, is the respiratory crisis. In addition to the lack, for now, of vaccine or medicine against its effects. Therefore, we see the high degree of virulence, the high mortality rate (particularly for elderly patients or those with pre-existing diseases) and the need for social isolation, which directly influence the economy. China, a country that initially presented a large number of cases in early 2020, needed to take severe measures towards social isolation. Among other factors, because the unprecedented nature of the disease was recognized.

An issue that appeared shortly after the mass manifestation of the disease is the situation of public health systems around the world. The neoliberal wave that has spread throughout the world in the last 40 years has disrupted or made unviable the structuring of universal health care systems in several national states. Although some resisted (such as the notorious British case), others (such as the Brazilian Unified Health System), even with the legal provision for universality, were left with less than necessary funding. Outside Europe, whose countries that have built a Welfare State have maintained reasonable health care, medical care is normally treated as a commodity. In general, the middle and upper classes use private health insurance, the best-known case being the US system. People with low purchasing power do not seek medical services due to high prices, or are served by low quality health insurance, with little coverage of services offered.

In a situation in which the need for supply of beds, in particular those in the Intensive Care Unit, is above normal, a major problem arises. Even those public health systems with good financing suffered strong demand, and this demanded that the contamination curve be "flattened," so as not to overload hospital beds in a short time. Hence the importance of policies of social isolation. In severe cases, even the adoption of *lockdown* in large cities. The figures presented regularly by the World Health Organization, since the pandemic character of the new coronavirus was recognized, point to a relative success of its containment in Asia. On the other hand, European countries that were slow to take restrictive circulation measures, such as Italy, were hit hard. The picture was unfortunately repeated in the United States and Brazil, whose presidents initially underestimated the severity of the disease.

One of the possible explanations for this behavior, considered by many analysts to be irresponsible, is that measures to contain the epidemic through social isolation directly affect economic activity. As a good part of the global economy, especially the western one, comes from years of low economic growth, the political leaders of these countries sought to avoid an even greater economic downturn. In the specific case of Donald Trump, the pandemic comes as he prepares to run for re-election to the presidency, in late 2020. Both he and Jair Bolsonaro, in Brazil, chose to use the speech of political hatred to maintain a social base support, but they did not have this contingency of nature.

Other questions also explain the behavior of both: the relationships they have with pharmaceutical companies. Trump is a shareholder in a company that produces chloroquine and hydroxychloroquine, drugs used to treat malaria and other diseases, which are under study as to whether they can be used for people infected with the new coronavirus. Even without scientific evidence regarding the effectiveness in this case, Trump has been trumpeting the use of these drugs, even without a prescription. In the case of Bolsonaro, the behavior is mimetic, and a businessperson supporting his government is involved with companies that produce these drugs. In addition, he ordered the Brazilian Army to produce a large amount of chloroquine, and now needs to dispose of the stock generated.

Neighboring countries, both in North and South America, fear that the behavior of the two countries will make it difficult to control the disease within their borders. The United States and Brazil are becoming the two major places of the disease in the world. In addition, the lethality of the disease shows that this situation is not only the physiological conditions of the people that lead for illness: social inequality in countries is also a risk factor. For social isolation policies to be successful, it is necessary for national governments to create policies to guarantee income and maintain jobs. In addition, the homes of people require a minimum infrastructure to ensure the hygienic conditions: sanitation, access to water etc.. Many countries in the West, especially those in America, is known for social inequalities and levels of poverty. The United States, despite its economic grandeur, has seen the percentage of people with precarious jobs, unemployed and homeless people grow significantly. Brazil is considered one of the most unequal countries in the world, although it is also a large economy. In both, not only is access to health systems precarious (in Brazil, at least, there is a universal system, even if underfunded), but income guarantee policies are very fragile. In these conditions, not only do poor people need to go out every day to try to earn some income, exposing themselves to public transport, but they also put people in their homes at risk, many without the necessary infrastructure.

Therefore, if we look at conditions prior to the start of the pandemic, it was possible to see a general increase in inequality, except in Asian countries that have experienced economic growth in recent decades. There is now a debate about the possibility, after the outbreak of this disease (which deeply shakes the economic dynamics), of more supportive and inclusive development alternatives. There are many approaches to the topic, from exaggerated optimism to nihilistic pessimism. Let us now seek to verify the possibilities and challenges for progressive and left-wing political forces around the world.

III. Seeking a more supportive world, bypassing adversity

First of all, we must recognize: the challenges that arise in the world during and after the COVID-19 pandemic will be enormous. Estimates of economic downturn vary between countries, but are expected to fall between -4% and -6% of the gross domestic product of national economies. In many ways, it is a situation similar to conventional long-term wars. Sporting and artistic events were postponed or suspended, as occurred during the outbreak of the two Great World Wars. The debate now taking place is about how economic reconstruction should take place.

The financial crisis of 2009, as we argued above, did not arise from the productive economy, and the action of the national central banks managed to contain the expansion of losses, which in any case were quite significant. As the mechanisms for controlling financial flows have not been profoundly altered, and the world economy seemed to show signs of some recovery, a part of the *mainstream* academic and conservative political forces began to advocate the resumption of fiscal austerity policies. Especially in the periphery of the system, policies more focused on national development, which seemed to be strong in the first decade of the century, were replaced by a new wave of liberal reforms. Already at the center of the system, notably the United States and European countries, parliamentary and presidential elections brought to power xenophobic and hostile proposals to countries of recent industrialization. Therefore, two obstacles emerged for policies to combat the pandemic and the resumption of world economic growth: refusal to make the State the driver of the economic resumption and aggressiveness in international relations, in the direction of a trade war.

Some analysts are betting that the economic crisis triggered by the pandemic may open the opportunity for new political arrangements. The realization that economic deregulation oriented towards self-regulated markets are dysfunctional is gaining more followers. Likewise, no economic recovery and no development strategy will be possible without state planning, combined with incentives to the private sector. Public investments in infrastructure (particularly in countries of recent industrialization), in addition to employment and income guarantee policies, will be required. A dynamic activity in the markets only occurs when the popular classes use their income for consumption, unlike the middle and upper classes, which tend to make financial investments with a good part of their income.

Since the COVID-19 pandemic will still require resources for health systems for a long time, it may be an opportunity for such services come out of strong market regulation. Access to health cannot be a commodity, but a public good. Many diseases do not choose social classes, and only a public and universal system can guarantee the control of diseases that may arise in the future – and they will certainly arise.

Providing public health systems also require efficient financing mechanisms. The most successful cases in the world indicate that this is only possible with progressive tax systems. The poor and recently industrialized countries tend to have regressive tax systems, whose taxes are more on consumption and lower income than on wealth and high incomes. Therefore, it will be necessary to face this issue in the different national contexts where a Welfare State has not yet been established.

What is indicated here for health systems is also valid for educational systems and national innovation systems: it will take a lot of investment to improve access to good quality schools and a good link between the public sector, private companies and academia. Since the resources required for such activities are enormous, it will be necessary to rethink the forms of international collaboration, for common purposes. Some countries have already adopted measures in this direction of international collaboration.

Cuba already has a long tradition of cooperation in the medical field, and this has been intensifying since the beginning of the pandemic. For example, sending doctors to European countries that have been hit hard by the pandemic, such as Italy. It also has *expertise* in the development of drug research, in collaboration with laboratories around the world. The President of the People's Republic of China, Xi Jinping, announced at a meeting of the World Health Organization in May 2020 that the fruit of efforts to develop treatment for COVID-19 will be shared with the entire world community. These are initiatives that can go a long way in reversing the individualism and the Hobbesian spirit of war of "all against all," which were very stimulated in the neoliberal globalization of the last decades.

This leads us to discuss, now, the perspectives for the international socialist movement. Everyone agrees that the end of the Soviet experience was a severe blow to the leftist forces, not only communists and socialists. Socialist countries that maintained their regimes, such as China and Cuba, were forced to face major limitations during the liberal offensive. However, paradoxically, globalization and the increase of economic ties of the different nations made it possible for the first time a global overcoming of the capitalist logic.

The neoliberal theses, which had been defended since the 1930s, had their concrete historical experience between the end of the 20th century and the beginning of the 21st century, and ended up demonstrating the limits of the so-called "self-regulated" markets. The unique way in which China was inserted in world trade, an economic opening combined with *catch-up* industrialization strategies resulted in a success recognized even by its opponents. Although the national characteristics of the People's Republic of China are unique, it's socialism with its own characteristics suggests that socialist regimes can use mechanisms to reduce poverty and erect a national development project.

What can be said for the moment is that neoliberal globalization has been deeply shaken by two events in just over 10 years: the subprime financial *crisis* and the productive crisis coming from the pandemic. What must happen now is a lack of definition in international geopolitics, which can be succeeded by retaining multilateral geopolitical systems, or rising tension arises from the military superpower, the United States. If we look at objective conditions, never in the history of humankind have there been so many opportunities to build a more rational, democratic and environmentally friendly system as now. There are significant cooperation efforts between networks of academic researchers, especially those in the health field, who were already active even before the start of the pandemic. Progressive and left-wing forces are strengthening ties on all continents, including to face the rise of neo-fascism in various parts of the planet.

IV. Conclusion

History has already taught us that material and cultural progress do not arise spontaneously. The possibilities that are opening up will not be realized alone. Socialist parties and forces, in their national contexts, need to come up with bold (but doable) proposals and engage in broad convincing activity. For, with the crisis of neoliberal hegemony, there was the rise of neo-fascism and extreme right parties. The easy speech of xenophobia and political hatred seems attractive to part of the workers.

National development projects, based on international collaboration between the "Global South" (countries of recent industrialization, such as those of the BRICS), are a real possibility, and were already outlined at the end of the first decade of the century. In national contexts, it will be necessary to implement infrastructure investment projects, creating an aggregate demand that makes it possible to increase the domestic product. This would make it possible to implement progressive tax policies, taxing large fortunes to finance education, health and Research & Development. The domestic markets of recently developed countries can be boosted with public investments in the private sector, conditioned by policies for job expansion. Public investment banks can foster solidarity economy activities, such as agricultural production cooperatives, which are essential for regional development.

The ways to increase national prosperity and international collaboration are possible and concrete. On the other hand, they constitute an immense challenge for world socialism. The more the capitalist market economy shows its deficiencies, the more necessary is the search for new paths. There is in fact a huge debate about the possibility of the Chinese model being a parameter for the construction of new forms of socialism. Nevertheless, the very existence of an alternative route to national development, which was not submitted to neoliberal canons, shows that this is plausible. Humankind's future depends on the ability to find such political solutions.

Prevention and Control of the Epidemic Highlights the Advantages and Disadvantages of Governing Capabilities of Socialism and Capitalism

[America] David M. Kotz

Edited by Zhang Li[1]

> **About the Author**
>
> David M. Kotz is a world-renowned Marxist economist. He is a professor of political economy at the Department of Economics in University of Massachusetts, vice-president of World Association for Political Economy, and a staff economist at Center for Popular Economics. He is a member of the Union for Radical Political Economics and a member of the Massachusetts Society of Professors.

China responded effectively to COVID-19 once the central leadership realized the danger it represented. The state was able to mobilize for an all-round response including locking down key areas; making sure people under lockdown had their basic needs met; rapidly increasing the capacity of hospitals and the production of protective equipment and medical supplies; doing a lot of testing; and monitoring

---

1   Zhang Li, associate research fellow of the Academy of Marxism, Chinese Academy of Social Sciences.

contacts with infected people. By the end of the March 2020, China had made important progress in prevention and control of the COVID-19 epidemic. However, the epedemic is spreading rapidly in the United States and other countries, and appears to be going unchecked at first sight.

The US federal government has had one of the worst responses of any country, as the President denied and minimized the problem for several months and then refused to have the federal government take over the response. This left states and localities to compete for scarce supplies. There has been no consistent policy. The president has refused to allow scientists to take the lead and has personally recommended dangerous products and actions such as injecting bleach into the body! Now the President is urging lifting the stay at home order before it is safe to do so. In Trump's administration competent officials have been systematically replaced by people who will praise Trump but have no useful skills, much like a Medieval king's court.

This difference between China's response and the US response is not entirely a matter of socialism versus capitalism. Some capitalist states have responded effectively, such as South Korea, New Zealand, and Denmark.

The bad response in the US is partly due to President Trump, who is both a right-wing nationalist and has serious mental health problems including narcissism (extreme self-love), inability to take responsibility under pressure, constant lying, and refusal to recognize reality. But even before Trump took office the US was not in a good position to respond to a pandemic, because decades of neoliberal transformation had weakened the US public health system, undermined the capability of government to carry out any difficult tasks, and encouraged a just-in-time production approach that did not build up necessary stocks of essential goods.

In general socialism is much better at responding to a pandemic than capitalism. A socialist planned economy is much better at a rapid reallocation of production to meet a sudden emergency. That is why the US government introduce central planning in 1942 after the US suddenly entered World War II – and it was very effective. A socialist system is oriented to meeting human needs, not pursuing profit, and that is the approach needed for confronting a pandemic. A pandemic creates a classical "public goods" problem in which everyone must be made healthy and safe regardless of ability to pay because anyone who gets infected will spread the disease to others. Capitalism is driven by pursuit of profit which runs counter to the approach needed to be prepared for, and to confront, a pandemic.

Some capitalist countries have had effective responses despite the problems of capitalism. That bears study. In some cases socialist ideas have influenced the state, as in Denmark and New Zealand. In some cases the state has a history of successfully managing the economy, such as South Korea. Germany has been relatively effective, and the German state has been influenced over time by the political power of the working class in Germany and the need for Germany to succeed in competition with socialist states to its east.

It is difficult to predict the effects of the pandemic on the US politics. So far it seems to be reducing support for President Trump and the Republicans in Congress, but it is too soon to be sure of the ultimate effect.

A World Changed by Novel Coronavirus

[Moldova] Mark Tkachuk

Edited by Chen Airu[1]   Translated by Li Yi   Finalized by He Jun

Abstract

The COVID-19 pandemic triggers the reflection on the transformation of state systems in the former Soviet Union and the countries of Eastern Europe. Following the collapse of the Soviet Union, the choices of state systems lead to economic recession and moral degeneracy in these countries, where the value of public health and the value of education are assessed from the perspective of economic efficiency. The COVID-19 pandemic is a "plume of

---

1   Chen Airu, associate research fellow at the Academy of Marxism, Chinese Academy of Social Sciences.

the historical balance" (i.e. measuring the good and evil in human nature) that demonstrates two paths of development in the contemporary world. It is apparent that the socialist medical system is more suited to responding to a pandemic. China's fight against the coronavirus provides the world with a clear example as to what kind of social system is on earth the most suitable one for responding to a challenge posed by an unconventional emergency in the 21st century. A new, clear global plan is unfolding, which will fundamentally expand employment and the demands supported by the capacity to pay, and establish an equitable social security system, public health system and education system with wide coverage. Only when all the countries and civilizations in the world are regarded as a unified community with a shared future, and the goal of global solidarity is promoted conscientiously, can humans get the upper hand in their fight against the COVID-19 pandemic, climatic disaster and economic crisis.

I. The COVID-19 pandemic triggers the reflection on the transformation of state systems in the former Soviet Union and the countries of Eastern Europe

Over the past 30 years, the countries located in the former Soviet Union and Eastern Europe always believe that the socialist legacies in the fields of economy, education, culture and sanitation and health care all lag behind the times, and should be mercilessly eliminated. Over these 30 years, these countries have implemented two kinds of systems based on their choices: the first represents a shift from the Soviet socialism to a market-based democracy in a transitional period of time; the second refers to more developed governance system, culture and civilization gradually evolved on the basis of a market economy.

The results from practice show that the first choice of system corresponds to a period characterized by economic recession and moral degeneracy. If some objectives have been achieved in this transitional period, they are obviously of no major social significance. The new powerful and rich people who account for only a very small percentage of the total population become the beneficiaries of this system, while millions of people are left behind. The truth is that the so-called "market economy" – if the state or the authorities fail to map out a strategy of orientation for social development – can only lead to a "market society," in which the most essential human values and cultural values – solidarity, sympathy, friendship between people, national dignity, and the health of the majority of the population (i.e. the elderly, the young, women and children) will all be turned into commodities and labeled with "reasonable" prices.

Therefore, the transition started 30 years ago did not replace the out-of-date socialism with a progressive and flexible path leading to capitalism, but brought the country back to a pre-capitalist system amid the crisis of the socialist system. Under the pre-capitalist system, the elites from the semi-feudal administrative organs in the post-Soviet Union period fulfilled their goal of theft by taking advantage of a barbaric market. A dispersed and atomized society is confronted with one challenge after another. In all the countries in the former Soviet Union, the market launched attacks year after year against science, education and health care by cutting the expenses on scientific research, canceling free education, and closing schools and hospitals. Since 2009, the Republic of Moldova has closed 300 schools and a large number of community-affiliated hospitals. Scientists, teachers, doctors and nurses have left their motherland in order to earn a meagre income abroad. The whole set of policies was called "optimization" policies by the government, and received the support from international financial organizations – the International Monetary Fund and the World Bank. The value that cannot be assessed by the market – the value of public health and the value of education – are assessed from the sensational perspective of economic efficiency.

The COVID-19 pandemic occurs along with the new round of crisis of capitalism. The COVID-19 pandemic is the trigger point rather than the root cause of the crisis of capitalism. All the defects of a dominating world order are exposed when it is confronted by this public emergency. The COVID-19 pandemic is a "plume of the historical balance" that demonstrates two paths of development in the contemporary world.

It is apparent that the socialist medical system is more suited to responding to a pandemic. For instance, the Semashko System (Николай Александрович Семашко) which was well known both at home and abroad during the period of the Soviet Union was proposed by Nikolai Aleksandrovich Semashko, people's commissar of public health, in 1924. Under the Semashko System, the funds were allocated under a unified budget, and the medical assistance was put under unified management. This model had been in operation until 1989. In addition, it was in the fight against large-scale epidemic diseases (the Spanish influenza, smallpox, cholera and tuberculosis) that the first free-of-charge public medical treatment model in the world – the Semashko System came into being in the Soviet Union. Based on proactive policies of preventing epidemic diseases, the Semashko System provided ordinary citizens with all kinds of medical services, and the entire system could rapidly and professionally mobilize resources in case of emergency. At present, not only the countries in the former Soviet Union but the EU member states (e.g. Italy and Spain) are reassessing the "optimization" policies that have been carried out in the public health system for decades.

Moreover, it is obvious that capitalist countries have failed to establish a medical and health care model whereby the majority of ordinary people enjoy the right to medical treatment on an equal footing. In particular, it is distressing that COVID-19 pandemic reveals the inconsistency between the values preached by the EU, where left-wing politicians and left-wing institutions traditionally hold sway, and the specific practices. For instance, as an EU member state, Italy was denied the solidarity and support of the whole of Europe which was of great importance to its battle against COVID-19 pandemic.

China's fight against the coronavirus provides the world with a clear example as to what kind of social system is on earth the most suitable one for responding to a challenge posed by an unconventional emergency in the 21st century. Moreover, we have witnessed the highest efficiency and the best results as well as the capability of rapidly mobilizing professional resources in China. China was the first country hit by the COVID-19 epidemic; it has also emerged a victor first in this formidable struggle, having brought under control the threat of the virus. China demonstrates that three cardinal principles should be adhered to in building socialism: first, pursuing benefits for the majority of people in the society; second, developing a public healthcare system that can constantly modernize itself and serve the ordinary people (rather than elites only); third, becoming a leader who can constantly improve the system of scientific knowledge.

II. The influences and changes caused by the COVID-19 pandemic to the world order

Probably many people have noticed the close relationship between epidemics and rebellions. The plague (also known as "Black Death") that occurred in France directly gave rise to the Jacquerie Uprising, the largest peasant revolt that broke out in 1358 and the 1381 Peasants' Revolt led by Wat Tyler in England. The epidemics costed the lives of nearly half of the population in Europe at that time.

Similar plague prevailing in Veliky Novgorod (Великий Новгород) from 1417 to 1420 led to the Novgorod Uprising (Новгородское Восстание) in 1418. We still remember the great famine and cholera that raged throughout the Grand Duchy of Moscow on the eve of its turbulence. While an epidemic was spreading, the Khlopok Rebellion broke out in the south of Rus (Русь).

The British revolution was closely related to the outbreak of typhoid fever and malaria. Today people believe that Oliver Cromwell, leader of the revolutionary troop as well as the independent faction, died because he unfortunately suffered from both epidemic diseases.

The Black Death plaguing Russia opened the prologue to the peasants' war led by Stepan Razin (Степан Разин) from 1670 to 1671. The epidemic spread throughout the whole country for 15 years prior to the outbreak of the peasants' uprising, sowing the seeds of hatred towards a regime comprised of men of property.

A large-scale plague broke out in 1771. After the epidemic subsided, a peasant uprising led by Pugachev (Емельян Пугачев) broke out in 1773 and lasted until 1775.

The cholera spreading from Sevastopol (Севастополь) to Moscow from 1830 to 1831 shocked Russia. In the same period, the November Uprising of 1830 broke out in Poland.

The outbreak of European Revolutions of 1848 was closely followed by the cholera epidemic in 1848. The smallpox epidemic in 1871 was a special result caused by the Franco-Prussian War, and it was followed by the founding of the Paris Commune. The Paris Commune disclosed a different kind of regularity which would be manifested in the 20th century.

The Spanish Flu Pandemic broke out following the end of the First World War. In the wake of the pandemic, revolutions erupted one after another throughout the entire Europe (Russia, Germany and Hungary); and uprisings and civil wars broke out in China, India and Egypt. The total number of deaths in the Spanish Flu Pandemic, the First World War and all revolutions amounted to at least 50 million.

The COVID-19 pandemic is a dramatic reflection of the global economic crisis. Both experts and politicians are unanimously saying that the world will never be the same. What they mean is that we will lose a large proportion of freedom we have taken for granted – the freedom of associating with other people, the freedom of international travel, and the freedom of personal life. Now, it is necessary to adopt entirely different standards regarding these freedoms. However, the paradox lies in the fact that most people in the world have never owned these kinds of freedom, and the majority of them are but bystanders attracted by freedom, and they are at most imitators of the "golden one billion"[1] who are able to choose the lifestyles they want.

Indeed, the world will never be the same. The global crisis raises an acute question: The economy based on the principle of "liberalism" cannot achieve further development; the "invisible hand of the market" seems to be unable to set long-term strategic objectives and plans. A new, clear global plan is unfolding, which will fundamentally expand employment and the demands supported by the capacity to pay, and establish an equitable social security system, public health system and education system with wide coverage. It is in this sense that there is the need to reassess the past socialist experience and the contemporary socialist path that China is following.

III. Coronavirus is an enemy to the whole of mankind, and its spread around the world highlights the important significance of developing a global community of shared future

The coronavirus is beginning to spread rapidly in Moldova. The virus has defeated the Moldovan government, as the number of infected cases per 100,000 people proves that Moldova is the "champion" of Europe, and this assertion is further substantiated by the daily infected cases and deaths. The Moldovan society is waiting for the effective measures against the COVID-19. However, the government and the Opposition in the parliament wasted the precious time when they deliberately made wrong choices. They concealed the fact that there was an outbreak of coronavirus cases in Hincesti (Хынчештский Район), and did not cancel the election campaign there. President Igor Dodon (Игорь Додон) and his team and Maia Sandu (Майя Санду) and her political group jointly established

---

1   "Golden one billion" refers to the one billion population living in developed countries. – *Chen Airu.*

an epidemiology center in Hincesti. It is no doubt both politicians should be responsible for what they have done.

Everyone has to play his/her role and undertakes his/her responsibility in political competition. Commanding political power – this is the administrative responsibility of primary importance. For the Opposition, the responsibility of first importance is moral responsibility. However, it is bad for the government to make this or that decision without undertaking moral responsibility. It is also bad for the Opposition to lose its sensibility and overstep the bottom line of human morality because of its crave for power.

The election should not have been held in Hincesti. In fact, many social activists angrily denounced the election, yet the election took place as scheduled. On election day, many philosophers commented that they saw real "political animals" (Политические Животные) in these politicians. The use of "political animals" makes people think that the expression refers to "real stinging and cold-blooded politicians."

It should be noted that there are a variety of animals. In addition to horses, dogs and cranes, there are worms, toads and mice. Listen to the loud shriek of the supporters of Maia Sandu who attempted to throw all the blames to the government, and look at the self-satisfaction of leaders of the Opposition who celebrated their victory in Hincesti in those sweet days, and you will understand that the rulers of Moldova are by no means the honest type like the horse and the crane.

The concept of "a global community of shared future" is no longer a declaration or a theoretical framework. The concept, as interpreted by Xi Jinping, president of the People's Republic of China, has won support of the United Nations and a number of international forums, including World Economic Forum held in Davos. Given the crisis of the COVID-19 pandemic, the concept of "a global community of shared future" expounds the necessity of establishing new partnerships of coordination among all countries with real cases.

Humans are extremely vulnerable when they are faced with a new type of challenge. On the one hand, the present international relations and international interaction exhibit vulnerability and instability. On the other hand, the spread of COVID-19 demands a change to the present world order. People should realize that a new type of relations between countries can be constructed only when the concept of "a global community of shared future" is used as a starting point. The new relations will see reduced use of violence, more empathy and compassion, and shared technology, information, expertise and wealth.

Only when all the countries and civilizations in the world are regarded as a unified community with a shared future, and the goal of global solidarity is promoted conscientiously, can humans get the upper hand in their fight against the COVID-19 pandemic, climatic disaster and economic crisis.

We Must Re-invent Europe

[Austria] Walter Baier

Edited by Li Xin[1] Yu Haiqing[2]

About the Author

Walter Baier is an Austrian economist. He was the chairman of the Communist Party of Austria from 1994 to 2006, and was an editor of the Austrian weekly *People's Voice (Volksstimme)*. He has served as the political coordinator of the network "Transform! Europe Network" since 2007.

Abstract

The COVID-19 epidemic reveals the sharp contradictions within the European Union and its structural flaws. The decline of European economy has become an undisputable fact. Since the outbreak of the financial crisis, the crisis of the European integration has always been a subject of the European policy. This stems from the conflicts between the market and democracy, because the integration of capitalist countries in their alliance is mainly realized through the market, while the market alone cannot satisfy the needs of society at large. The reshaping of Europe in the post-corona era calls for

---

1　Li Xin, doctoral candidate, School of Marxism, Shandong University.
2　Yu Haiqing, research fellow of the Academy of Marxism, Chinese Academy of Social Sciences.

> the long-term and resilient supranational cooperation. The Leftists need to link the resolving of the epidemic crisis with social-ecological transformation, and develop a new strategy on the cracks that the crisis in public discourse has opened up. The pandemic and the global ecological crisis demonstrate that neoliberalism's world market project has failed as a civilizational model, and highlight the importance of strengthening international cooperation. Europe needs to propose a realistic solution based on people's interests. Exploring the new forms of China-Europe communication and cooperation will provide an opportunity for constructing a world characterized by peace, equality and solidarity at a higher level.

Prediction is very difficult, especially if it's about the future.

It is a widely held view that the COVID-19 crisis has ushered in a new era. We share this view to the point that it is difficult to imagine that the world could return to the status quo ante. It will not. However, our thesis is that the pandemic has not caused but rather accelerated the critical factors, which will determine the global developments in the years to come. This applies in particular to the world system in which unilateral US hegemony is coming to an end . The attempt to present this from the perspective of Europe and its integration process is the goal of this contribution.

On December 31, 2019, China had informed the WHO of the occurrence of "pneumonia of unknown cause" in Wuhan. On January 12, China was sharing the full genome sequences of SARS-CoV-2 with the international platform GISAIR and the WHO.

Hence, when the health ministers of the EU member states met in Brussels on February 13, they had sufficient information to react but failed taking preventive measures against the pandemic's spread. Subsequently, those countries, whose healthcare systems had been emaciated by decades of austerity policies were left alone with the rapidly spreading disease.

While the European Central Bank (ECB) mid of March reacted to the looming crisis with a bond purchasing program of 120 billion Euro, the finance ministers of the EU countries agreed only on a temporary suspension of the Fiscal Compact, which means they delivered a temporary solution to problems that would not at all exist if it were not for the Fiscal Compact.

The flagship project of the EU the free movement of people granted by the Schengen Agreement was abolished, however, not due to a decision taken collectively to provisionally close borders but because of the individual uncoordinated decisions taken by European governments.

At the beginning of March, Germany even blocked the export of protective medical equipment, which not only made a mockery of European solidarity, but rather violated the otherwise sacrosanct domestic market rules.

Thus, the coronavirus crisis has exposed the crass contradiction of the EU treaties assigning social and healthcare policy to the member states but constraining their financial bases by EU legislation – primarily the Growth and Stability Pact (Fiscal Compact). It is doubtful that the damage this has done to the EU's prestige, especially in the states most tragically affected by the epidemic, can still be repaired.

The existential crisis, in which the EU now finds itself is mercilessly revealing its structural flaws: the wrong prioritising of the European treaties – whose main concern is not the wellbeing of the populations but the unobstructed functioning of the markets – and the wrongheaded division of competences between the EU institutions, which substitutes the principle of the democratic, parliamentary formation of will at the national levels with a non-transparent interaction between governments and the EU bureaucracy on the European level.

At the time of writing of this text, it seems that the acute phase of the pandemic is over in the European Union. Almost all states have lifted restrictions on the freedom of movement of citizens and the decommissioning of public life, including large parts of the economy. True, there are fears of a resurgence of the plague in autumn and winter, but what now enters into the centre of concern is the beginning of the economic crisis about whose extent and duration nobody can be sure. Reputable economists are warning that it could be the biggest economic crisis capitalism has yet seen in peacetime. With its economic governance and the prevailing neoliberal, economic supply-side doctrine, it is reasonable to think that the EU is ill prepared to protect Europeans from its effects.

What ought to be the hour of European solidarity threatens to become "a Walpurgis Night on the nationalist Bald Mountain,"[1] the moment of the radical right which already now tries to capitalize on the crisis by escalating its aggressive discourse.

However, the nationalist idea that a crisis of global dimensions can be solved by nations competing with each other for scarce resources is completely irrational, above all for the small and medium-sized states of the EU. The more the absurdity of the nationalist view becomes obvious the greater will be the temptation to authoritarian methods of rule. The path from illiberal democracy to dictatorship may now prove to be a short one.

We are already now seeing the political and cultural backlash, which is expressing itself in the increase in domestic violence and in the displacement of women from public discourse, paradoxically at a time when work in care and reproduction, which today is mainly performed by women, proves its systemic importance.

The European Left needs to face the seriousness of the situation. Capitalism is coming up against its systemic limits. Yet if this statement is to serve as anything more than ideological self-affirmation, we need a debate about the alternatives that Europe's people now face and the possible paths to a new mode of production and culture.

I. How will Europe face the recession?

Recession of Europe's economy is already a fact. What is not known is

---

1   Luxemburg, Rosa: *Fragment über Krieg, nationale Frage und Revolution*, p. 367 f.

whether it will lead to a longer-lasting depression. The last financial crisis, despite the victims it claimed, did not lead to the collapse of capitalism; rather, the richest percent of the world's population was able to push its levels of wealth to undreamt of extremes, and, via the financial markets, it now has the populations and states more firmly in its grasp than ever.

The current recession, by contrast to the previous one, is not triggered by a collapse of the hypertrophic financial sector but from an abrupt break in the supply and demand sides and the value chains of the real economies.

In theory, one could imagine a kick-start of the economies after the end of the pandemic's acute phase and a quick return to normality. What speaks against this is the fact that the real economy, burdened by geopolitical tensions, was already in a downswing before the pandemic. The attempts by central banks to use expansive monetary policy to stimulate investments and real economies is correct but it is doubtful that it will be lastingly effective.

Above all, however, in view of digitalisation and the environmental crisis, the capitalist economies are at the threshold of a comprehensive transformation that requires strategies other than those contained in neo-classical economics textbooks.

Meanwhile, unemployment rates have reached dramatic heights. According to International Labour Organization (ILO) 2.7 billion workers have been affected by partial or full lockdown measures globally. The social time bomb in Europe, created by the millions of temporary labour relationships, unprotected by labour laws and social rights is now in danger of exploding.

To pre-empt the immediate social and economic effects of the lockdown, governments have passed special programmes of a hitherto unheard of scope, for example the German government is incurring to finance a package of measures decreed at the end of March, amounting to 10 % of GDP. Economists are expecting a rise in debt levels in relation to the GDP of the Eurogroup members by 10 to 15 percentage points.

While the European Commission limited itself to ex post legitimising the decisions taken by states, in contrast at least the ECB acted by indicating its readiness to buy up state bonds at a total value of 750 billion euros. This can provide a temporary relief.

At the end of May, it finally became obvious that the impending crisis could turn into an existential threat to the EU and the integration process as such, and that it cannot be dealt with solely by means of excessive monetary policy, but required robust fiscal stimuli, which in turn could not be left to the member states alone.

EU Commission President Van der Leyen presented a European development plan ("Next Generation EU") of 750 billion euros. When this text was finalized, it was still controversial among the member states as to how this program should be financed and in what proportions it should consist of subsidies to countries particularly affected by the crisis or of repayable loans, which, would only be available under restrictive austerity conditions. This however is repudiated by the countries concerned, whose sovereign debt already now exceeds any sustainable level and would be augmented if they were forced to new borrowings. Thus, without a big hair cut the course is being set by today's coronavirus crisis for tomorrow's state debt crisis and austerity policy. The effects of debt accumulation hit countries obviously very differently, since the interest rates give an advantage to the financially powerful states and discriminate against the weaker ones.

The effect is striking: Germany accounts for 50% of the amounts spent so far by the member states to deal with the consequences of the crisis, even though its share in the EU economy is only 26%. Thus, indebtedness will further aggravate inequality between the deindustrialized regions in Southern and Eastern European and the economic power centres of the EU.

Yet, some important things remain unpredictable. The economic structural transformation will alter the position of industries, regions, and states within capitalist competition and change their financial clout, will add new contradictions and rivalries to the already existing East/West and North/South fault lines which may even affect the core of European integration.

Additionally, the economic reconstruction after the end of the acute phase of the pandemic, which must be linked with the ecological transformation of the industrial and energetic basis of the economies, will demand unprecedented investing. The financing of private and public debt, which is again growing exorbitantly during the crisis, will therefore become the key problem of the post-corona period. Coming up with an answer to this is the most important task the left now needs to face.

In this context, the debate about the European mutualizing of borrowing which came up already during the financial meltdown 2007 remerged. The idea is that through Eurobonds, the joint financial strength of Euro-group members could be deployed to create low-interest loans, making them available to the states in proportion to how affected they are by the pandemic and the subsequent economic recession. The proposal's brusque rejection on the part of the German government however throws a dark shadow over the future of European integration in the post-corona era.

Eurobonds could provide relief, but the general problem of the states' high debt levels and their negative effect on the division of material and political resources among the states and classes will persist unless a radical haircut on the European debt and a change in the distribution of resources and income would be achieved.

The financing of state debt through inflation would meet fierce political opposition in some of the EU member states, particularly in Germany. The alternatives then are either to unload the burdens onto the populations through austerity and privatisation programmes, as in the last crisis, or to make the owners of great wealth, who hold the lion's share of loans, themselves bear the interest burdens of public budgets through debt forgiveness, confiscatory capital levies, and a capital gains tax.

Carrying out such a policy will need to be accompanied by imposing capital controls and by guaranteeing the claims on capital-funded pension and health-insurance funds, which should be accomplished by the public sector's takeover of these funds, which must be enacted by the member states, however supported and coordinated on a supranational level.

In the coming months even mainstream economists will not tire of assuring us that they were never neoliberals. The Left can build on the cracks that the crisis in public discourse has opened up. However, we have learned from the last financial crisis that this window of opportunity will remain open only until a consensus forms within the ruling classes, mainly of the large European countries, on how to deal with the crisis. Therefore, the left should avoid becoming the left wing of the liberal mainstream. This is not about a doctrinal contest. The crisis is posing the question of hegemony regarding the social interests that should be crucial in dealing with it.

Although temporarily ousted from the public discourse, the epochal challenge posed by the ecological crisis remains. An alternative in the interests of the majority of the populations has to link the solution of this acute crisis to socio-ecological transformation. The decisive criterion is not to reach an agreement among broad circles on general goals (this already exists) in Europe but on the tools needed to implement them. What is at issue is the institutions and the balance of power between classes. We must have the courage to talk about a new role of the states, about property, about the socialisation of the financial sector, about capital controls, about economic democracy and the strengthening of wage dependents at the level of enterprises, municipalities, countries, and the EU. This is the only way in which we can take advantage of the opportunities to expand social space for a new hegemony.

II. The Market-Democracy-Dilemma

At the end of 2019, the European Commission and the European Parliament indicated that a Conference on the Future of Europe involving citizen participation is promised. With reference to the pandemic, the start of this process has been postponed indefinitely.

The theme of the crisis of integration has occupied European policy since the financial crisis. In 2017, the European Commission published the White Paper on the Future of Europe. The five scenarios for the future of the EU, exposed in this paper whose main author has been the then president of the Commission Jean Claude Juncker meanwhile fell into oblivion. In September of the same year, at the Sorbonne, French President Emmanuel Macron announced in a keynote address the "Initiative for Europe," in which he called for the abolition of unemployment, an ecological transformation, a financial-transaction tax, a digital tax, the establishment of a minimum rate of wealth tax, the convergence of social standards, a clear increase in the EU's budget, and the democratisation of EU institutions. Macron omitted none of the EU's deficits in calling for a "refoundation of Europe!"[1] But, only a little later, when the heads of the German and French governments met in Paris for the 55th anniversary of the Élysée Treaty for the friendship between France and Germany, the closing statement contained nothing of Macron's proposals. And so the debate had already come to a standstill before the European Parliament elections.

The "flagship projects" on which it was possible for the Member States to reach an agreement were the armament programmes and the expansion of Frontex – the European Border and Coast Guard Agency. Military spending and defence against refugees are apparently always feasible, while the completion of the banking union, which implies a financial obligation on the part of the large banks to fund a European Deposit Insurance is put on hold. Also disappointing this year, in its scope and mode of financing, was the European Green Deal, through which the Von der Leyen Commission intended to react to the climate crisis.

The EU's failure in social and climate policy should not be surprising since the integration of capitalist states in a union cannot occur other than primarily through markets, which have no feel for society-wide needs.

---

1   "Sorbonne speech of Emmanuel Macron (English version)," see http://international.blogs.ouest-france.fr/archive/2017/09/29/macron-sorbonne-verbatim-europe-18583.html.

The EU milestones – the Treaties of Rome, the Single European Act, the Treaty of Maastricht, and the Treaty of Lisbon – have continuously deepened the EU's market-economy character. And even Emmanuel Macron, in contrast to his aforementioned innovative gesture in his keynote address at the Sorbonne, has called the domestic market "the real soul of Europe."

However, integration via markets had, from the very beginning, been opposed by a social countertendency based on the priority given to centrally planned political decisions taken by the European institutions to embed economy within policy goals by means of state and supranational institutions. Indeed, the history of European integration can be accounted as the clash of these two tendencies.

The European Coal and Steel Community was founded in 1951, replacing the International Authority for the Ruhr, which after the War had placed West Germany's heavy industry under Allied control. Alongside trade in the products of heavy industry without customs barriers, a High Authority was created with far-reaching dirigiste powers.

The "politics-market" conflict reached a climax in 1984 when the first directly elected European Parliament accepted the Draft Treaty establishing the European Union written under the guidance of Altiero Spinelli. It provided for the European market economy's subordination to social targets – explicitly named as full employment, the overcoming of inequality, protection of the environment, and cultural progress. Moreover, the initiative in the shaping and further development of the union was to be shifted to the European Parliament – and without restricting the rights of the national parliaments.[1]

What followed was completely different to Spinelli's aspirations. In 1985 the heads of states and governments passed the Single European Act, which set the goal of quickly realising an all-encompassing European internal market, which signified

---

1   "Draft Treaty establishing the European Union," February 14, 1984, see https://www.cvce.eu/ en/obj/draft_treaty_establishing_the_european_union_14_february_1984-en-0c1f92e8-db44-4408- b569-c464cc1e73c9.html.

the victory of the market-economy tendency. In 1992, when the heads of states and governments met for the summit at Maastricht after the situation of the world economy and geopolitics had fundamentally changed following the establishment of neoliberalism and historic events of 1989, they felt confident to complete this victory through the creation of an economic and monetary union with the now famous criteria of "convergence."

The conflict flared up again in 2005 when the heads of states presented their new construction, a draft of the Treaty for Establishing a Constitution for Europe, for ratification by the populations of all member states and were rebuffed in three countries. That the failed constitution was passed by an intergovernmental conference two years later as the Treaty of Lisbon bypassing popular ratification, certainly did nothing to improve the EU's standing.

The most recent dramatic climax in the battle between market and democracy came in 2015 when Syriza, having come to government in Greece, sought to break out of the straitjacket of neoliberal austerity policy.

The harshness with which the attempt to find an alternative way out of the crisis was quashed by the creditors and the brutality of the austerity programmes forced on it – much harder to those imposed to Ireland and Portugal – horrified many throughout Europe; but it also reanimated the differences in attitude towards the EU that had always existed within the radical left.

The question, which the European Left, along with the lefts of each country, has to answer, which scale and form of European cooperation or integration, different to the present EU, it sees as appropriate for confronting contemporary capitalism. The answers will vary depending on whether the focus is Europe as a whole or the individual states, and depending on each country's situation.

The right of countries to leave the European Union or the Eurozone is incontestable. Despite the growth of disintegrative tendencies, a disorderly breakup of the EU in its 27 or more components, at least under conditions of peace, is a rather improbable scenario. More plausible would be a re-emergence of old lines of conflict in Europe between a Central European bloc under the aegis of Germany and a Southern and Western bloc led by France. It is doubtful whether this new kind of order can lead to more stable social and political relations.

It is a fact that in many countries the longstanding disillusion with the European Union has evolved into a conviction that it is not "reformable." We cannot ignore this change of mood nor try through compromise to conceal the differences in how the EU is perceived, since it constitutes a point of departure for the strategic debate that now needs to take place.

If the strategic task is to recover the sovereignty of the peoples not against each other but together in the face of the financial markets, then the democratic self-determination of the populations and their control of their states have to be defended. This implies the right of every progressive government to disobey those rules which hamper the wellbeing of their states and societies. We must therefore demand that the Growth and Stability Pact, inactivated during the coronavirus crisis, should not come back after its end, but be abrogated. Instead of it, the EU's financial instruments – the ECB, the European Investment Bank, and the European Stability Mechanism – must be available to finance national programmes to reconstruct the healthcare and social systems and, beyond this, the ecological transformation of the economies.

The strengthening of the social infrastructures, the reconstruction and ecological transformation of Europe's industries, the elimination of regional disparities, the building of effective energy and transportation nets, with the mobilisation of the necessary financial capacity reaching beyond the scope of the current EU budget – all this requires long-term and resilient supranational cooperation. If this is not to be left to the markets, it also needs a rather close supranational political cooperation.

The left should build a strategic project for this cooperation. Today the EU is present as a strange hybrid: on the one hand a free-trade and single currency zone with a bureaucratic apparatus, which proved incapable of action in the crisis; on the other hand a parliament that does not have the power to manage the market and bureaucracy.

This leads to the question of political leadership. Europe's left needs to be active also on the European political scene as a power that stakes a claim to leadership. A claim to political leadership requires conducting a struggle for the expansion of democracy. The argument of the liberals – that the deficit of European democracy consists in the lack of a European public opinion – is weak. It is more accurate to say that European civil society, the trade unions, and social movements only have limited capacities to influence European policy, for which the decisive factor still is, apart from the structural neoliberal and non-democratic characteristics of the EU, dependent on the hierarchy of its member states as determined by their relative economic and political weight.

It is in a way trivial to say that the left's essential power bases are located in the nation-states. Protecting them from the destructive tendency of the uncontrolled market economy is strategically necessary in any case.

Therefore it is crucial to emphasize that in all conceivable systems of European cooperation/integration the states continue to be economic and political powers in their own rights and will remain so for the foreseeable future; this needs to find expression in a transparent and efficient system of defined jurisdictions and checks and balances between them and the Union.

However, since political developments in the individual states proceed at different paces and influence European developments to different degrees, the excessive weight of the national governments in European policy acts as a filter that obstructs social changes. This produces the stalemate we are in.

The only way to overcome the stalemate is through the diffusion of democracy to all levels of decision-making, which means that it is also at the European level at which diverse and antagonistic parties need to compete for influence, cooperate with each other, or confront each other.

As a step in the long process for the refoundation of Europe, based on a post-capitalist vision, this requires, a sovereign, freely elected parliament interacting with the trade unions, the social, ecological and civic movements. In place of the European Council comprised of heads of state and governments, the European Parliament must become the centre of the decision-making in those affairs for which the EU has authority. In it the key factor would be the intervention of political parties at the European institutional level. The Party of the European Left should seriously examine to advocate their upgrading by asking them to run for the elections of the European Parliament with European lists.

III. The dilemma of Pan-Europeanism

Brexit will not only change the life of the 3.5 million EU citizens within the UK and the 1.2 million UK citizens living in the EU Member States but the EU as a whole.

UK has been EU's third biggest national economy and one of the five "official" nuclear powers holding a permanent seat in the UN Security Council. The fact that it parallel negotiates a far reaching free trade agreement with the US spells out the geopolitical dimension of Brexit. The emphasis primarily on trade and competition which the EU lays in the negotiations seems the latter not sufficiently taking into account.

The European Commission arrogantly is counting on the UK's economic dependency on the EU greatly outweighing the EU's on the UK. Yet, this alone does not tell us anything about the Commission's actual negotiating strength.

The UK side has also a big problem: it is interested in the continued unobstructed access of British financial services companies to the EU market. This will involve concessions to the detriment of other sectors in Britain, for example fisheries, which will not be easy to achieve. In addition, exit from the EU is aggravating the disintegration tendencies within the UK, with Scotland thinking seriously to hold a referendum on its independence and then rejoin the

EU, something that will fuel existing separatist tendencies in other parts of Europe. At the same time, the danger of revival of hostilities in Northern Ireland cannot be underestimated since it is not impossible that Brexit could put in danger even the Good Friday Agreement.

The treaty on UK-EU partnership, whenever it will be established, must undergo a complicated process of ratification by the European Council, the European Parliament and Britain's Parliament. It is possible that its ratification by the national parliaments of EU Member States will also be required. The process can extend far into 2021 and beyond.

The left certainly favours a fair and just deal between UK and EU. It is not certain that the negotiations will be successfully concluded. If they collapse amidst mutual accusations, this will only benefit the nationalists on both sides of the English Channel.

UK's exit from the EU can reminds us once again that pan-Europeanism is not confined by the borders of the actual EU. We have to think about the really existing European Union in a new way.

The EU is not a universal European entity and will not be one for the foreseeable future. Therefore, and not only due to its obvious deficits, it cannot claim a monopoly on the issue of Europe's cooperation/integration. Thus, it is misleading to think the "finality" of the EU as a continuously expanding state on the model of the US. Latest the defeat of EU's strategy in the Ukraine should have demonstrated the dangers of such a model of gradual expansion.

IV. Europe's place in the world

The pandemic has made clear that the most dangerous threats facing societies are not military but social and ecological, which is gradually but increasingly understood by the people all over the world.

Protection from military aggression is in the first place a political task consisting in the strengthening of international law and cooperative structures. The creation of new nuclear weapons of mass destruction resulting from the abrogation of the Intermediate-range Nuclear Forces Treaty (INF Treaty) on the part of the US and Russia and the imminent expiration of the Strategic Arms Reduction Treaty (START Treaty) represent a continuing danger to Europe.

The end of the arms race and the management of the ecological crisis require international cooperation on a global scale, in which Europe has to redefine its role. This also requires the reanimation of those European forums that have disappeared behind the European Union in the public's perception: the United Nations Economic Commission for Europe, the Council of Europe and the Organization for Security and Co-operation in Europe, to which all states on the continent belong.

The pandemic and the global ecological crisis demonstrate that neoliberalism's world market project has failed as a civilizational model, and has cost human lives not only in the global South but also in the developed world, including Europe. Yet, the necessity of a global transformation hits the barriers of a political and military world order being in turmoil itself. In this context, we must interpret Donald Trump's presidency far more as consequence, than as cause of the crisis in US hegemony.

Whilst the US president in a blame game tried to distract from the failures of his administration in responding to the sanitary crisis, and accused China for a lack of cooperation, the *Financial Times* reported about the ongoing collaboration of US scientists with their Chinese colleagues in investigating the origin of coronavirus. Soon later, the US-president directed his anger even against the WHO with which he seized to cooperate.[1] The European Union has to define its position in this expanding field of tension.

Ironically, at the very moment when the outbreak of the pandemic in Europe

---

1   "US and Chinese researchers team up for hunt into Covid origins," *Financial Times*, April 27, 2020, see https://www.ft.com/content/f08181a9-526c-4e4b-ac5f-0614bf1cffb3.

underlined the importance of enhanced international, the EU Commission attempted to, at least verbally, accommodate itself to the aggressive tone from the other shore of the Atlantic, by declaring China to its "systemic rival."

To be clear about it, we are far from pleading in favour of taking uncritical stances towards China and each of its domestic and external international moves. Neither does the very diverse European Left, which upholds the value of democratic socialism, look at China as sort of ideological role model, which it would follow in a completely different context.

However like it or not, China is not only the most populous country in the world, it is after the US the EU's biggest trade partner. Let alone all the political and military dangers inflicted by it, the US-president's confrontational politics, imperils also global trade and global cooperation in dealing with the ecological crisis.

Thus, Europe requires a realistic approach based on the interest of its populations. China is a world power, which has also influence on Europe. The EU should, the Cooperation between China and Central and Eastern European Countries (China-CEE, 17+1 format) involving both members and non-members of the EU in a dialogue, perceive not as a threat, but rather as a form of international cooperation providing new and interesting political and economic opportunities.

The EU-China summit originally planned for autumn in 2020 under the German EU Presidency and postponed due to the Corona-Crisis should not be a diplomatic event but could be also an occasion to discuss in a broader public how the relations between these two powers can develop in the interest of a more peaceful, equal and solidary world.

COVID-19 and Governance Issues

[India] Srikanth Kondapalli

Edited by Zhang Shulan[1] Le Qing[2]

About the Author

Xie Gang, whose original name is Srikanth Kondapalli, is a professor of Chinese studies at Jawaharlal Nehru University in India, and a specially-invited commentator for Indian media. He has been regularly quoted by BBC news, *China Daily, The Atlantic, New York Times, Indian Express, The Guardian, Times of India, Wall Street Journal, Washington Post* and Xinhua News Agency.

---

1   Zhang Shulan, researcher of South Asian Studies Center and Institute of Contemporary Socialism, Shandong University.

2   Le Qing, graduate student of Shool of Political Science and Public Administration, Shandong University.

Abstract

COVID-19 spread across China and the world reflects to a major human tragedy, and it in all likelihood will go down in human history as one of the most decisive events. China adopts stringent measures to check the spread of the epidemic, while actively providing medical assistance to other countries affected by the epidemic. China makes strenuous and timely efforts in conducting international cooperation. Facts prove that the existing organizations of the international community are incapable of effectively responding to coronavirus, and that new and more effective multilateral measures need to be adopted. The COVID-19 pandemic has exerted huge impacts upon public health, the economy and social development, and has potential influences upon regional and global order.

COVID-19 spread across China and the world reflects to a major human tragedy with over 300,000 deaths and suggests to the limitations in human endeavour to address natural diseases and pandemics which have grown world over. Since late 2019, a highly pathogenic novel Coronavirus, now renamed as Coronavirus Disease – 2019 (COVID-19 in short), spread to most parts of the globe within no time – thus affecting billions of lives, their health and wealth[1]. In its trail are millions of patients across the globe, hundreds of thousands of deaths and turmoil and dislocations all around. By the end of May 2020, according to the World Health Organization estimates, there are over 6 million infections of COVID-19, over 363,000 deaths in 216 countries. The worst affected today include the American Continents, Europe and other developing countries. COVID-19 also disrupted on a large scale as well travel, transportation networks, economies and the political systems. Despite advances in scientific knowledge and medicines, as with

---

1   See the State Council Information Office of the People's Republic of China, "Fighting COVID-19: China in Action," *Xinhua*, June 7, 2020, see http://www.xinhuanet.com/english/2020-06/07/c_139120424.htm.

the other strains of Coronaviruses, COVID-19 did not witness the development of a vaccine yet, thus complicating millions of lives across the globe. China and the world literally came to a standstill for several days, weeks and months as nation after nation resorted to complete or partial shutdowns, enforced quarantines and unforeseen restrictions on travel as the contagion spread to the nooks and corners of the world. In the recent living memory, no other disease has had so much of negative impact on the humanity. China's Premier Li Keqiang encapsulated the problem in his speech to the National People's Congress on May 22, 2020 that COVID-19 "is the fastest spreading, most extensive, and most challenging public health emergency" since the People's Republic of China (PRC) was established in 1949.[1] This applies to other countries as well.

Thus, COVID-19 in all likelihood will go down in human history as one of the most decisive events in terms of its global scale, the unprecedented fear that it generated across vast swathes of the world, the kind of economic destruction that it inflicted across the board, barring a few sectors (such as pharmaceuticals, environment etc.) and for the comprehensive dislocation it brough about, including in the regional and global orders. An estimated four billion people are in some form or the other of lockdown in the nooks and corners of the world so as to break the chain of contagion.

I. Outbreak of COVID-19

According to various studies, COVID-19 was broke out in Wuhan and spread to the Hubei Province followed domestically. The Spring Festival rush – the annual family reunions for hundreds of millions of Chinese – further aggravated

---

1   Li Keqiang, "Premier Li's speech at the third session of the 13th NPC," *CGTN,* May 22, 2020,see https://news.cgtn.com/news/2020-05-22/Full-text-Premier-Li-s-speech-at-the-third-session-of-the-13th-NPC-QHaP1FpB8k/index.html.

the situation by spreading the virus.[1] An estimated 3 billion trips are made in such family reunions posing grave danger in spreading the contagion.[2] However, due to community isolation, the areas that are far away from Hubei province did not witness COVID-19 infections such as in Inner Mongolia Autonomous Region, Tibet Autonomous Region and Qinghai Province.[3] In later period, COVID-19 spread to the north-eastern Heilongjiang province with suspected infection spread from a foreign returnee.

Given the intensity of the transmission of COVID-19, China had undertaken strict measures to contain the contagion. The Chinese government adopted a five-level response to counter the spread of the COVID-19 as follows:

1. regional isolation measures in Wuhan by shut down on January 23,

2. concentrates on the temporary isolation and,

3. rescue hospital construction – Leishenshan and Huoshenshan,

4. organizes the medical staff of all Provinces from China to support Wuhan in improving their treatment capacity so as to rapidly digest the backlog of suspected cases and,

5. reduce the number of viral infections by blocking community transmissions and introducing mobile phone applications like "Shen I" and "Health Code".[4]

Thus, it is only two days after the lockdown of Wuhan that on January 25 a small leading group was formed by the central leadership of the communist party. According to the Emergency Response Law of the PRC, which is implemented on November 1, 2007, the Premier of the State Council is made responsible to address

---

1   Ye Jiachen, Hu Qitong, Ji Peng, and Marc Barthelemy, "The effect of interurban movements on the spatial distribution of population in China," March 16, 2020, see https://arxiv.org/pdf/2003.07276.pdf.

2   Wang Hairong, "An All-out War," *Beijing Review,* February 13, 2020,see http://www.bjreview.com.

3   Hu Zixin et.al., "Artificial Intelligence Forecasting of Covid-19 in China," March 1, 2020, accessed at https://arxiv.org/ftp/arxiv/papers/2002/2002.07112.pdf.

4   See Zhou Yimin et.al., "The Outbreak Evaluation of COVID-19 in Wuhan District of China," accessed at https://arxiv.org/pdf/2002.09640.pdf.

"emergencies."[1] The small leading group was tasked to visit Hubei and coordinate and "to treat infected patients, speed up the augmentation of medical personnel, and coordinate civilian and military medical resources."[2] Premier Li Keqiang was named the head of this group (who visited Wuhan on January 27[3]), with other members including Vice Premier Sun Chunlan[4] (who is in charge of the health sector). Premier Li also directed replenishment of doctors and nurses from other provinces and nearly 43,000 personnel were rushed to Wuhan later.[5] On January 28, meeting the visiting World Health Organization chief, President Xi stated that "The epidemic is a devil. We will not let it hide."[6] President Xi Jinping addressed the armed forces stating the situation in "grim and complicated."[7] In all 14 Politburo Standing Committee meetings took place from January till May – indicating to the apex political leadership's unprecedented concern on the issue. Two hospitals to cure patients were being constructed at Wuhan and over 43,000 medical personnel

---

1   See "Emergency Response Law of the People's Republic of China," November 1, 2007 at http:// english.mee.gov.cn/Resources/laws/envir_elatedlaws/201705/t20170514_414040.shtml. Article 3 of this law states that "emergencies include natural disasters, calamitous accidents, public health accidents and public security incidents, which occur abruptly and cause or may potentially cause serious social harm and for which measures for handling emergencies need to be adopted."

2   See "CPC leadership meets to discuss novel coronavirus prevention, control," International Department of the CC of CPC at http://www.idcpc.org.cn/english/events/202001/t20200127_137500. html.

3   During the visit, Li stated that "we must fight resolutely to win the battle against the epidemic." See "Chinese premier in Wuhan, demands all-out efforts in epidemic prevention, control," Xinhua, January 27, 2020 at http://www.xinhuanet.com/english/2020-01/27/c_138737735.htm.

4   Sun served in Fujian and Tianjin as party secretary. She reshuffled the health organisations in China by establishing National Health Commission in March 27, 2018 which is to cover "comprehensive, lifecycle" issues of health in China. She visited Wuhan extensively for medical relief operations.

5   See "Premier Li visits medical staff in Wuhan," January 28, 2020 at http://english.www.gov.cn/ premier/news/202001/28/content_WS5e2f871ec6d019625c60408e.html and "So Long, Farewell," Beijing Review, March 26, 2020 at http://www.bjreview.com.

6   "Xi Jinping meets with visiting World Health Organization (WHO) Director-General Tedros Adhanom Ghebreyesus," January 29, 2020 at https://www.fmprc.gov.cn/mfa_eng/zxxx_662805/ t1737014.shtml.

7   "Unremitting efforts," Beijing Review, March 5, 2020 at http://www.bjreview.com.

from across the country were sent for medical relief purposes. President Xi visited Wuhan on March 10. By April 8, China declared that Wuhan and other areas have not reported fresh cases of COVID-19 and testing of a majority of the population is being undertaken extensively. While some asymptomatic cases were reported, the numbers of fresh infections are under control.

Outside China, the first COVID-19 case was reported in Thailand first on January 8 and confirmed on January 14. Another case was reported in Japan with the cruise ship *Diamond Princess* reporting many cases later when it was docked off Yokohama. The earliest cases of infections in Italy were traced to January-February period, two cases tested positive at Rome on January 30, while on February 3 a group of 56 Italian tourists arrived at Rome and among whom one tested positive on February 6. On February 20, the first case of COVID-19 was reported in Lodi in north-western Italy. A majority of cases were reported in Italy from three regions – Lombardy, Veneto and Emilia-Romagna.[1] COVID-19 now further spread to 216 countries in all, with the worst affected in North and South Americas and Europe. Significantly, it is re-emerging in many countries and other parts of the world, despite the enormous testing and preliminary medication. Asymptomatic cases and mutation of the virus are said to be on the rise. These suggests to the limitations in human understanding of the nature, science and technology capabilities and responses to control the pandemics.

II. COVID-19 and International Cooperation

Despite these limitations, a number of countries came forward to address COVID-19 for vaccine development or supply of immediate medical necessities on a national and international scale. In the light of the spread of COVID-19 across the

---

1   Diego Giuliani, Maria Michela Dickson, Giuseppe Espa, and Flavio Santi, "Modelling and predicting the spatio-temporal spread of Coronavirus disease 2019 (COVID-19) in Italy," March 23, 2020 at https://arxiv.org/pdf/2003.06664.

globe, the necessity to pool together scientific knowledge, experience and medical expertise and equipment across the world has become imperative. The United Nations and its institutions such as World Health Assembly and World Health Organization are providing significant alerts to the international community about the spread of COVID-19.

China's response in international response is at two levels – one of supporting multilateral efforts and second assistance or supplies of medical equipment to the COVID-19 affected countries.[1] Overall, China announced provision of medical aid in medical equipment (gloves, masks, personal protection equipment, testing kits and others), technological cooperation (medical personnel, video conferences, etc.), sister cities cooperation with counterparts across the world and NGOs or enterprises support (such as Alibaba's donations etc.).[2]

Early on Beijing organized, in the immediate neighbourhood, an online Eurasian and South Asian virtual meeting of health officials to coordinate their efforts. President Xi addressed the G-20 leaders virtual meeting that took place on March 26 under the leadership of Saudi Arabia. China suggested "information-sharing, strengthen cooperation on drugs, vaccines and epidemic control, and cut off cross-border infections."[3] On May 13, 2020, the Shanghai Cooperation Organisation held an online conference that stressed the centrality of the UN system in addressing COVID-19. President Xi Jinping, in his address to World Health Assembly on May 18, 2020 announced $2 billion in assistance to the developing

---

1   For a list of President Xi Jinping's speeches in this regard, see "Xi Jinping: Unity and Cooperation Are the International Community's Most Potent Weapon to Overcome the Pandemic," April 29, 2020 at http://en.theorychina.org/top_2475/202004/t20200429_368587.shtml.
2   See "Foreign Ministry Spokesperson Geng Shuang's Regular Press Conference on March 20,2020" at https://www.fmprc.gov.cn/mfa_eng/xwfw_665399/s2510_665401/t1758992.shtml.
3   "What China has done to boost int'l cooperation against COVID-19," *Xinhua,* May 17, 2020 at http://www.xinhuanet.com/english/2020-05/17/c_139064005.htm.

countries in addressing the COVID-19 fallout.[1] Besides, according to a Xinhua report, China provided "anti-epidemic supplies to more than 150 countries and international organizations, held over 120 video conferences with more than 160 countries and international organizations, and sent 21 teams of medical experts to 19 countries."[2] According to Zhang Ming, China's representative to the European Union, China is to support the COVID-19 ACT Accelerator programme launched by the World Health Organization and work with Coalition for Epidemic Preparedness Innovations (CEPI), GAVI (the Vaccine Alliance) and other international agencies in terms of pharmaceuticals, vaccine and testing.[3]

The International Monetary Fund announced $1 trillion in assistance to its 189 members and pledged to cancel debt scheduling payments to 25 countries for half-a-year invoking the Catastrophe Containment and Relief Trust provisions.[4] European Union and other countries committed $8 billion in funds for further research and development of medicines and vaccines to counter COVID-19.[5]

There are also specific international collaborative projects worth mentioning at the bilateral level. In the early stages of the COVID-19 outbreak at Wuhan and other places, several nations have come forward with medical assistance. Most notable of these was Japan's gesture of donation of medical equipment by invoking a classical

---

1   See "Xi Jinping: Fighting COVID-19 Through Solidarity and Cooperation Building a Global Community of Health for All," May 19, 2020 at http://en.theorychina.org/top_2475/202005/t20200519_368638.shtml.

2   "Fighting COVID-19 Through Solidarity and Cooperation Building a Global Community of Health for All," May 18, 2020 at https://www.fmprc.gov.cn/mfa_eng/zxxx_662805/t1780221.shtml.

3   "China to expand COVID-19 cooperation special fund, says envoy at global pledging event," *CGTN*, May 5, 2020 at https://news.cgtn.com/news/2020-05-05/China-to-expand-COVID-19-cooperation-special-fund-says-envoy-QeFnoKhY76/index.html.

4   Masaya Llavaneras Blanco and Antulio Rosales, "Global Governance and COVID-19: The Implications of Fragmentation and Inequality," May 6, 2020 at https://www.e-ir.info/2020/05/06/global-governance-and-covid-19-the-implications-of-fragmentation-and-inequality/.

5   "Global leaders promise $8 bln to fight COVID-19, EU says," *CGTN*, May 5, 2020 at https://news.cgtn.com/news/2020-05-04/EU-to-provide-1-bln-euros-for-global-vaccine-search-QdYYwCnp3W/index.html.

saying "Although we are in different places, we are under the same sky."[1] In March, India provided China with 15 tonnes of medical equipment when an Indian Air Force transport delivered these supplies at Wuhan.

China as well supplied medical equipment and sent personnel to the affected countries as the virus spread. In vaccine development, China's CanSino Biologics Inc. made a tie up with Canada's National Research Council for future trials. Earlier, China exported 32 tonnes of medical equipment to Canada to fight COVID-19.[2]

To the United States as well as to the South American countries, China has sent supplies of ventilators, testing kits, masks, gloves, PPEs and others.[3] During Ebola virus crisis, China sent over 1,000 medical workers and provided Yuan 750 million to the affected countries. To address the COVID-19 cases, China sent medical teams to Ethiopia and Burkino Faso. As president Xi Jinping stated: "Five Chinese medical expert teams have also been sent to the African continent. In total, in the past seven decades, over 200 million people in Africa have received care and treatment from Chinese medical teams. At present, 46 resident Chinese medical teams are in Africa helping with COVID-19 containment efforts locally."[4] Towards West Asia, China's medical assistance to Iran has been noted given the massive spurt in COVID-19 cases initially at Qom and other places. China also sent medical relief supplies to Turkey, Iraq and Palestine, and collaborated with Israel on medicine. To other regions such as South Asia, Southeast Asia and others, China's efforts at cooperation is considerable and timely.

---

1   "Japan offers warm support to China in battle against virus outbreak," *Xinhua,* February 13, 2020 at http://www.xinhuanet.com/english/2020-02/13/c_138779612.htm.
2   "China confirms cooperation with Canada on COVID-19 vaccines, drugs development," *Times Now,* May 14, 2020 at https://www.timesnownews.com/health/article/china-confirms-cooperation-with-canada-on-covid-19-vaccines-drugs-development/591635.
3   "Fighting COVID-19 requires international cooperation," *China Daily,* April 2, 2020 at http://ex.chinadaily.com.cn/exchange/partners/45/rss/channel/www/columns/419cf7/stories/WS5e8ec473a3105d50a3d1504d.html.
4   "Fighting COVID-19 Through Solidarity and Cooperation Building a Global Community of Health for All," May 18, 2020 at https://www.fmprc.gov.cn/mfa_eng/zxxx_662805/t1780221.shtml.

III. COVID-19 and Global Order

The outbreak and spread of COVID-19 to different parts of the world and the death trail, loss of economy, supply chains, travel, tourism, cross-border movements, crash in energy prices and the like have all resulted in its far-reaching impact on the global and regional orders. Famously mentioned by American strategic expert Henry Kissinger, COVID-19 had ushered in a new order.[1]

Since the outbreak and spread of COVID-19 to many parts of the world, death toll and misery continued, the existing institutions proved to be inefficient to tackle the virus. The traditional models of global governance are based on a trend in the western liberal internationalism which suggested to intensifying institutional cooperation. One of the proponents of this view, James Rosenau in the volume *Governance without Government* famously mentioned about global governance for "purposive behavior, to goal-oriented activities, to systems of rule… refers to activities backed by shared goals that may or may not derive from legal and formally prescribed responsibilities."[2] Subsequently, John Ruggie proposed that "governance, at whatever level of social organization it may take place, refers to conducting the public's business: to the constellation of authoritative rules, institutions and practices by means of which any collectivity manages its affairs."[3]

---

1   "The Coronavirus Pandemic Will Forever Alter the World Order," *Wall Street Journal,* April 3, 2020 at https://www.wsj.com/articles/the-coronavirus-pandemic-will-forever-alter-the-world-order-11585953005. See also Kurt Campbell and Rush Doshi, "The Coronavirus Could Reshape Global OrderChina Is Maneuvering for International Leadership as the United States Falters," *Foreign Affairs,* March 18, 2020 at https://www.foreignaffairs.com/articles/china/2020-03-18/coronavirus-could-reshape-global-order and Thomas L. Friedman, "Our New Historical Divide: B.C. and A.C. — the World Before Corona and the World After," *New York Times,* May 17, 2020 at https://www.nytimes.com/2020/03/17/opinion/coronavirus-trends.html.
2   James N. Rosenau, "Governance, Order and Change in World Politics," in James N. Rosenau Ed. *Governance without Government: Order and Change in World Politics* Vol. 20: Cambridge Studies in International Politics (Cambridge: Cambridge University Press, 1992) p.4
3   John G. Ruggie, "American Exceptionalism, Exemptionalism and Global Governance," in Michael Ignatieff Ed. *American Exceptionalism and Human Rights* (Princeton, NJ: Princeton University Press, 2005) p.307

More prominently, Robert Keohane and Joseph Nye argued that governance is "the processes and institutions, both formal and informal that guide and restrain the collective activities of a group."[1]

In the backdrop of the ineffectiveness of many international institutions currently, the United Nations Security Council was tasked to address pressing security issues of the world. Yet there has been no positive and effective momentum in this regard. The World Health Organization remained only advisory in nature and clearly with funding cuts from member states, even such functions are going to be affected. The other institutions such as G-7, G-20, IMF and World Bank or Asian Development Bank as well did not make much difference, although the Bretton Woods institutions have put on hold the debt payments from developing countries. The G-7 foreign ministerial meeting on March 25 failed to come out with a statement, divided as it were by the name of the virus. Much of this paralysis in the current international institutions is traced to the emerging "decoupling" or "great power competition" between the two largest economies in the world, the United States and China.[2] With active recriminations against each other increasing, many an international body proved to be ineffective in tackling COVID-19. This suggests to the need for new but more effective multilateral responses from the international community.

Even as the economic growth rates for most countries has been slashed by the International Monetary Fund and other credit rating agencies, dwindling exports and imports due to lack of demand caused by general lockdown in many countries (with

---

1   Robert O. Keohane and Joseph S. Nye, "Introduction." in Joseph Nye and John Donahue Ed. *Governance in a Globalizing World* (Washington, DC: Brookings Institution Press, 2000) p.12

2   Zhang Yuyuan argued that the previous "one superpower, many major powers" ("一超多强" 格局) has undergone transformation. One of the effects of globalisation is the large scale of trade that flourished but also China became its main beneficiary. With nationalism and protectionist trends in the US, COVID-19 adds to the uncertainty in this trade supply chains. Zhang argued that the existing multilateral institutions would be transformed. See Zhang Yuyuan, 《新冠疫情与国际关系》 ("Novel Coronavirus epidemic situation and global pattern"), 《世界经济与政治》, April 2020 at http://www.doc88.com/p-14459450304223.html.

the World Trade Organisation estimating double-digit decline in trade), disruption in supply chain, curbs on travel and tourism, energy prices fluctuations and others have caused near economic depression conditions. Global debt has surpassed over $2.5 trillion according to the IMF estimates. Individual countries have announced monetary and fiscal stimulus packages but these appear to be inadequate to address the global decline. Unemployment in formal and informal sectors is staring at many countries due to COVID-19 lockdown. There has also been 40% decline in foreign direct investments globally. If the aggregate demand and supply issues are not addressed at the global level, if the US-unilateralism is not addressed quickly, and if the 2nd and 3rd waves of COVID-19 infections increase, humanity is expected to face major economic problems in the near future. It is estimated to it's about lose over $8.5 trillion in goods and services production in 2020, a gap that could hardly be filled up even in rebound conditions. These suggests to the need for intensifying macro-economic coordination efforts. Of course, many countries tried to utilize S&T innovation, big data, artificial intelligence, cloud computing and others to tackle the COVID-19 crisis but that also calls for new business models.[1]

In relation to China, many scholars see the post-COVID-19 world order as providing opportunities, specifically in international cooperation efforts. Yan Xuetong argued that while the international system is prone to several setbacks as well as inter-state conflicts, and despite the "decoupling" with the US, it is likely to strengthen globalization process. Yan suggested that COVID-19 does not have the capacity, like the World War II, to change the international pattern.[2] On the other hand, Yang Jiemian

---

1   Yoichi Funabashi, "Time to build the post-pandemic world order," *The Japan Times,* June 9, 2020 at https://www.japantimes.co.jp/opinion/2020/06/09/commentary/world-commentary/time-build-post-pandemic-world-order/#.XuHD8OR7nIV.

2   See Yu Xiaoqing, 《疫情会永久性改变世界秩序吗？》(Will the epidemic permanently change the world order?), 澎湃新闻 , April 29, 2020 at https://www.thepaper.cn/newsDetail_forward_7194686 Yan suggested that the US leadership handling of the epidemic has costed it its leading role in the world. Song Xiaoling, 《阎学通：新冠疫情不会对世界格局产生根本影响》 ("Yan Xuetong: Covid-19 will not have a fundamental impact on the international pattern"), 世界和平论坛 at http://www.sss.tsinghua.edu.cn/publish/sss/8393/2020/20200411211002811944109/20200411211002811944109_.html.

termed the current situation as a "qualitative inflection point" (质变拐点) in the emerging balance of power in the international system with reduction in the US power and enhancement in China's influence in World Bank and the IMF, Climate Change, WHO etc.. However, Yang argued that process of change will be slow.[1] Cui Hongjian of China Institute of International Studies is circumspect in that COVID-19 has brought about a kind of stalemate and the future depended on changes in "boosting or watershed" (助推器还是分水岭) elements.[2] Writing in *Global Times* Li Haidong argued that the spread of the epidemic will result in global economic crisis, leading to a remodelling of the current international relations. Li suggested that those countries which have high health safety measures and environmental protection mechanisms will become the leader of the new form of globalization in the post-COVID-19 order. The effective addressing of the epidemic control would also translate into "legitimacy of international behaviour" (国际关系行为的正当性), favouring China.[3] For Wang Yiwei, due to the superiority of the Chinese system and its efficient response mechanism, it is not only prepared to construct a "Silk Road of Health" but also prepare for positioning in the international system by enhancing its RMB circulation, overcoming the US threats to relocate its industries from China.[4]

The above discussion suggests that as COVID-19 spread across it brought innumerable problems never seen by the humanity in recent memories. It impacted

---

1   Yang Jiemian, 《大疫背景下的国际战略格局变动》 ("Changes in the international strategic landscape in the context of the epidemic"), March 30, 2020 at http://www.siis.org.cn/Research/Info/4910.

2   Cui Hongjian, 《疫情对世界格局变化的双重作用》 ("The dual effect of the epidemic situation on global pattern change"), 《国际问题研究》, April 30, 2020 at http://www.ciis.org.cn/gyzz/2020-06/08/content_41178069.htm.

3   Li Haidong, 《疫情深刻改变国际关系格局》 ("The epidemic profoundly changes the pattern of international relations"), 《环球时报》, March 31, 2020 at https://opinion.huanqiu.com/article/3xdewES5D3V.

4   Wang Yiwei, 《新冠肺炎疫情如何影响国际格局？专家解读7大方面，两项直接关系中国》 ("How does the novel Coronavirus epidemic affect global landscape – Expert interpretation of 7 major aspects, two directly related to China"), 《环球》 杂志, April 1, 2020 at https://www.jfdaily.com/wx/detail.do?id=232181.

on public health, economy, society and exhibited potential consequences for the regional and global orders. China argued through its recent white paper that its efforts to prevent and control COVID-19 have been efficient, timely and transparent. Since February China also had singled out international cooperation as a way out of the large-scale destruction that has occurred and articulated such position in multilateral processes.

Romania in a Tangled Warfare in 1989 and the Global "Health War" in 2020

[Romania] Constantin Crețu

Edited by Yu Haiqing[1] Li Ming[2]   Translated by Li Yi   Finalized by He Jun

---

About the Author

Constantin Crețu was born on October 17, 1949 in Romania.

From 1969 to 1972, he was the chairman of the College Students Federation of the Chemistry Department, University of Lasi.

From 1992 to 1996, he served as a member of the National Council of the Social Democratic Party of Romania.

From 1996 to 1998, he was a deputy chairman of the Romanian Workers' Party and head of its International Liaison Department.

From 1998 to 2003, he was a deputy chairman of the Romanian Socialist Party of Labor and head of its International Department.

From 2003 to 2008, he was a founding member of the Socialist Alliance Party, and served as its deputy chairman and head of its International Department.

From 2004 to 2008, he was a founding member of the Party of the European Left, a member of its Executive Committee, and a member of the Collaboration Committee of the Party of the European Left and São Paulo Forum.

---

1   Yu Haiqing, research fellow of the Academy of Marxism, Chinese Academy of Social Sciences.
2   Li Ming, research fellow of the International Department, Central Committee of the CPC.

From 2010 to 2012, he was a founding member and deputy chairman of the Reconstruction Committee of the Romanian Communist Party.

From August 8, 2012 to June 27, 2016, he served as the chairman of the Organization and Registration Committee of the Romanian Communist Party.

On June 27, 2016, the Romanian Communist Party – 21st Century was registered, and Constantin Crețu served as its founding chairman.

Abstract

"Romanian Communist Party – 21st Century" is a Communist organization newly founded in 2016. Constantin Crețu, chairman of the Party, wrote an article reviewing the historical reason for the failure of the Romanian Communist Party, with the focus put on the history of Romanian socialism and the tortuous process of reconstructing socialism after 1989.

He believes that in the present "health war" raging through the world, coronavirus, the invisible enemy having nothing to do with nationality, ethnic group or belief, ruthlessly attacks all countries in the world. To avoid the spread of coronavirus, we need, first and foremost, to reduce the flow of people between countries. Seen from this perspective, Romania is in a disadvantageous position. Romanian Communist Party – 21st Century believes that the NATO should be reformed to adapt to the realities of a changed world and eventually move towards self-disintegration in accordance with a global defense agreement involving countries like China, Russia, India and Iran.

April 17, 2020 marked the 31st anniversary of the Ninth Congress of the Grand National Assembly of the Socialist Republic of Romania. On this day I recalled the words of Nicolae Ceausescu, president of the Socialist Republic of Romania: "Just as I said at the plenary session of the Central Committee of the Romanian Communist Party convened on March 4, 1989, for the first time in its history of more than 1,000 years, Romania does not have any foreign debt, nor does it pay tribute to anybody any longer. Romania is indeed independent politically and economically." There is no political independence to speak of without economic independence. Our achievements in paying off debts and developing socialism were closely linked with the policies of the Romanian Communist Party, and they were the result brought about by the Romanian Communist Party that resolutely applied scientific socialism to the realities of Romania!

However, the fact that Romania cleared all foreign debts ran counter to the wishes of global financial imperialism, who made preparations to launch a propaganda campaign against Romania and eventually destroyed socialism in Romania and the rest of Europe by bringing down their national economy. It took them US$1.5 trillion to do all these. Later, based on a carefully fabricated lie, they labelled all the national leaders who would not bow to global financial imperialism "dictators," drove them off the political stage, and had them sentenced to death just as what they did to President Nicolae Ceausescu. On his way to the execution ground, Ceausescu shouted at the top of his voice: "Long live the free and independent Socialist Republic of Romania! History will avenge me!"

From December 2 to 4, 1989, Mikhail Gorbachev, president of the Soviet Union and American President George H.W. Bush held a meeting at Malta, at which Bush persuaded Gorbachev to trade ideological security for economic security. However, economic security has never been realized. Both leaders also agreed that the US can interfere with the affairs of Panama, and remove President Manuel Antonio Noriega from power. Meanwhile, with the support of President François Mitterrand who acted on behalf of the NATO, Gorbachev engineered a military coup carried out by the special troop in Romania. This coup, which was later called a "revolution," was aimed to remove President Ceausescu from the state leadership of Romania.

Saint John Paul II was the only person who predicted the disastrous aftermath of the understanding on the European socialist system reached between Gorbachev and George Bush Sr. from December 2 to 4 in 1989 in Malta, and he gave a warning. On the eve of the meeting in Malta, Saint John Paul II personally told Gorbachev: "The changes should not be made too rapidly. It is wrong for anybody to proclaim that the changes of Europe and the World should follow the Western model. As a participant of the world history, Europe must breathe with both of its lungs."

It was for this reason that in his letter to Mikhail Gorbachev on November 27, 1989, Nicolae Ceausescu said, "We think it is wrong and beyond understanding to propose de-ideologization in handling state-to-state relationship. Our Party believes that the ideology cannot be thrown away in international relations so long as imperialism exists."

Such a stance of the Romanian leader at the end of 1989 is substantiated by American President Donald Trump's approach (who publicly proclaimed to "remove" the leadership of the Communist Party of China in China) and the behaviors of the American Senate and leaders of other capitalist countries. They shift the blame to China and take actions to "sue" China for the so-called "reason" that China "produced" this virus worldwide. Such a stance is further proved by the worldwide anti-communist stance of preventing the Communist Party from emerging and launching activities over the past 30-odd years.

Today, 31 years on from the military coup occurred in December 1989, we see how Romania has turned from an internationally recognized medium-developed socialist country in which outstanding achievements in every field were achieved, including free education and medical care for the people, into an imperialist colony in the international community since it became a member of the NATO in 2004 and a member of the EU in 2007. The losses Romania has suffered total more than US$3 trillion. Romania's national industry and agriculture have been destroyed, its mineral resources plundered and owned by multinationals; more than 45 percent of arable land has been sold to foreigners, and more than 6 million Romanians are forced to go abroad to look for jobs. The majority of education and public health sectors is privatized. Following the instructions of the EU, more than 140 hospitals are dissolved, with medical workers forced to go abroad to look for jobs.

As a NATO member that has an established military partnership with the US, Romania is forced to pay two percent of its gross national product as armament expenses; with its own funds, it has set up and supported military bases for the permanent stationing of American troops, and has sent troops to the battlefields opened by the American troops.

The privatization implemented in Romania in an attempt to become a member of the EU effectively brought an end to its socialist industry and agriculture for good. "Returning everything to private ownership" damaged national interests: the country's natural resources were sold to multinationals, investment plans were cut, and Romania was turned into a country exporting cheap labor to developed capitalist countries.

Meanwhile, Romania has lost its decision-making power as a sovereign state after establishing military strategic partnership with the US. With respect to its diplomatic and economic policies, Romania follows the instructions of ambassadors of the US and major capitalist countries of the EU who are stationed in Romania. This is also the reason why Romania has been declined to join Schengen for many years. Although Romania has satisfied all the requirements raised by the EU, it still cannot become a signatory of the contracts signed between the EU and China each year. Its attempt to participate in cooperation in the areas of the economy and trade and infrastructure under the framework of the Silk Road has not been a success.

Faced with such severe internal and external environments, Romania cut the numbers of hospitals at the request of the EU. As a result, large numbers of high-caliber medical workers have left Romania. Those in power are indifferent to maintaining and equipping state-owned hospitals and staffing them with needed medical workers. In the current outbreak of the "health war," coronavirus, the invisible enemy having nothing to do with nationality, ethnic group or belief, ruthlessly attacks all countries in the world.

It is obvious that to avoid the spread of coronavirus, we need, first and foremost, to reduce the flow of people between countries. Seen from this perspective, Romania is in a disadvantageous position. The reasons are that out of more than 6 million Romanian citizens working abroad, more than 2 million do not have labor contracts, are not covered by medical insurance, and do not own personal houses or unemployment relief. The majority of them have already or will return to Romania soon.

Romania's request for help from Germany, which included the provision of necessary medical equipment and supplies, was rejected. In early April 2020, when Romania did its best to respond to the epidemic, the Romanian government issued a military order which required all Romanian residents to stay at home. However, at the request of Germany, more than 90,000 Romanians were sent to Germany to pick asparagus, regardless of the dangers they will encounter there.

The EU has also adopted differentiated treatment towards its member states. It has provided €300 billion to Germany and France for fighting coronavirus, while it has provided merely €2 billion to Romania for the same purpose.

It is known to all the unemployment rate of Romania has been the envy of other European countries over the years. According to formal statistics, the unemployment rate of Romania has always remained far below five percent. However, these reports reflect only part of the facts, because most people with working capacity opted to get employed in developed EU countries since they cannot find jobs in their own country. In fact, as Romania "exports" unemployment, it is hard to see true unemployment data in Romania from the statistics.

The present problem facing us all is that Romania has no funds at all to support any domestic economic activities, because multinationals have taken the lion's share of the profits. In the budget plan for 2020, economic development accounts for only one percent of GDP. It can be therefore concluded that it is colonialism and financial imperialism rather than coronavirus that have destroyed the life of the Romanian people. At present, Romania is burdened with foreign debts exceeding US$100 billion; by contrast, in March 1989 Romania had no foreign debts at all.

With the discovery of a more effective method of fighting and stemming COVID-19, a serious economic and food crisis begins to appear. This requires a new way of handling international relations, or in other words, letting solidarity and collaboration play a bigger role, rather than conducting unfair competition and interfering with the internal affairs of other countries. It is necessary for Romania to restore its sovereign status at a higher speed so that it can manage economic and social development on its own.

People are increasingly aware that Romania is not becoming stronger after its accession into the NATO. Instead, the national security is becoming more vulnerable than ever. Romania has become a potential target of the confrontation between Russia and the US and its allies, and the attack of terrorist organizations.

Romanian Communist Party – 21st Century holds that the NATO should be reformed to adapt to the realities of a changed world and eventually move towards self-disintegration in accordance with a global defense agreement which should involve countries like China, Russia, India and Iran. In this sense, Romanian Communist Party – 21st Century dedicates itself to a policy that will bring Romania back to its traditions rather than adopt the present proactive policy, so as to realize the denuclearization in the Black Sea and the Balkan Peninsula. Efforts should be made to enable Romania to enjoy an active neutral position and to secure the guarantee from the People's Republic of China, the Russian Federation, the United States and the United Nations to replace its membership in the American military strategic axis with its membership in an economic strategic axis. Romania must develop its relations and collaboration with major world economic powers based on principles of mutual benefit, no interference with internal affairs, and respect for Romania's independence, sovereignty and territorial integrity.

The problems facing Romania when it joined the EU should be ascribed to not only a lack of strategic vision at some time during the negotiation, but also the stupidity, incompetence, cowardice and even betrayal of those in power in Romania. We failed to obtain the assurances of fully respecting our immediate interests, failed to stand on an equal footing with others in transferring resources and receiving compensations, and failed to ensure that these resources would be used for the common good. We even made concessions, and are still paying a heavy price for these concessions.

Here we first point out that Romania accepted the policy of "deindustrialization" when it became a member of the EU. However, Romania did not receive real compensations through the integration policy following the pre-set specific schedule after it joined the EU. Later, the judicial department of Romania was brought under the control of external forces. As a result, the anti-corruption battle has lost its fixed goal – eliminating corruption, but has been reduced to becoming a political tool used to eliminate the elites in political, economic, administrative, academic and military fields in Romania.

Due to their subservient attitude, some Romanian leaders have turned Romania from a partner, collaborator and ally of the EU into its vassal state ever since the country's accession to the EU. These leaders surrender Romania's national interests in exchange for foreign support so that they can pocket the wealth left by new colonists who plundered Romania. Therefore, we will not forget the mistakes made by Romania leaders in power when criticizing foreigners who promote their own interests without paying more attention than we do to protecting the interests of Romania. Therefore, Romanians – I will not speak of Romania, because I have no idea whether she still exists or who she is – have every reason to complain that they are inferior citizens in the eyes of the EU.

The program of the "Romanian Communist Party – 21st Century" stresses that we are dedicated to building a Europe comprised of independent, unified national states with sovereignty, a Europe without double standards, and a Europe that can ensure all its member states to develop on an equal footing. Germany and France are advocates of European countries developing at different speeds. Given that situation, Romania has not been approved to join Schengen Area, nor has it avoided the MCV examination yet, although it has been an EU member country for 13 years. In addition, some people with tarnished image have been promoted to leaders of the EU without the consent of Romania. All these are reasons why the sovereignty movement of Romania is gaining momentum, to which our Party gives encouragement and support.

Outline Interview: Socio-economic Formation and the Fight Against COVID-19

[New Zealand] Katjo Buissink

Edited by Song Lidan[1]

About the Author

Born in 2000, Katjo Buissink is the chair of the Central Committee of the Communist Party of Aotearoa[*] in New Zealand. While he lived in Sydney, Australia during his childhood, he participated in the activities of the Communist Party of Australia (CPA). After returning to New Zealand, he led the reconstruction of the Communist Party of New Zealand, and recently graduated from Victoria University of Wellington. He has written articles and pamphlets about Marxism and trade unions, such as *Eco-Socialism or Eco-Imperialism?: Two Roads for the Environmental Movement, Why Does the Communist Party Have a Policy of Peace?* and *An Introduction to Community Unionism: Theory and Practice.*

[*] Aotearoa is the pronunciation of New Zealand in Maori.

---

1   Song Lidan, associate research fellow of the Academy of Marxism, Chinese Academy of Social Sciences.

Abstract

The response to COVID-19 draws stark contrast between socialism and capitalism. Different values manifested as "serving the people" and "putting profit first" lead to different results in epidemic prevention and control. As the pandemic will have important impacts on the global landscape, the US foreign policy will likely get more desperate and erratic as its dominant position in the world is further replaced by cooperation and non-alignment. Unity in struggle of world anti-imperialist & peace forces is the keystone in the struggle against interventionism and for the human community of a shared future.

I. The response to COVID-19 draws stark contrast between socialism and capitalism

The People's Republic of China's response to COVID-19 highlights the superiority of the socialist system in caring for the needs of citizens. To put it simply, under socialism working people are the politically dominant class and this is shown in the effectiveness of the socialist "China model" in epidemic control. An entirely new virus of this significance is the ultimate public health challenge for any country, and therefore growing pains are to be expected while a response is developed. What is important is the speed and dedication of the response.

The effectiveness of the Chinese response to COVID-19 can be seen in the insanity of the propaganda put out by anti-China forces in the West as time goes on. These anti-China forces have been unable to maintain a consistent story about why they dislike China's response, which highlights its actual strength.

To start off with, before COVID-19 spread throughout the West, they cried that the lockdown and similar measures to control the spread of the virus were "authoritarian" and unnecessary. Once their own countries were overcome by COVID-19 on a scale far worse than China, they changed their lies entirely to claim that China "had lied about the virus" and not done enough to control it! The fact that anti-China forces have had to lie so brazenly highlights the strength of the Chinese response, a fact mirrored by unbiased groups such as the World Health Organization.

China was the most severely affected country in the world at first. The Chinese government have taken the most stringent measures. In less than 2 months, China managed to control the spread of the epidemic and won precious time for other countries in the world to fight against this epidemic.

I think it is the socialist system allowed China to have such an excellent response, particular because of effort in recent decades to strengthen the rule of law and socialist democratic system. The unity of the people of all ethnic groups and the people-dedicated nature of the government, Communist Party, and People's Liberation Army (PLA) are absolute treasures of the Chinese socialist system.

Look at the incredible work of the People's Liberation Army running hospitals and playing such a vital part in the public health response. During the Civil War and War of Resistance against Japan, the people's army served the people against military aggressors, but Comrade Mao Zedong also emphasised the role of the people's army in peaceful production. In the present era of relative peace, the People's Liberation Army has served the Chinese people through public health. It is impossible to imagine any capitalist army in the West having such a dedication to the people and peace. Anti-China forces try to claim that the PLA seeks military conquest of the world. How can they try to justify this when the PLA's main activity has been peacefully running hospitals and protecting people's health?

The grassroots-based Chinese political system has also been incredibly important. The neighbourhood temperature checks, quarantine system and food delivery has allowed for greater self-isolation than in the West. China's socialist system allows for self-isolation and quarantine measures to be very effective, while in most Western countries working people have been forced to carry on almost as normal due to needing to work, buy groceries, etc..

At the end of March, China has achieved important initial results in controlling the virus. However, the epidemic has spread rapidly in the United States and other countries, without being controlled in the first place.

The United States is the centre of modern imperialism and the creator of the "Washington Consensus" that has wreaked havoc across the world. It is no surprise that this country is the hardest hit by the COVID-19 pandemic, as public health measures are not something the US Government is familiar with. You cannot invade a virus nor provoke a colour revolution within it. In recent years, the US has even used public health programmes as cover for military operations abroad. Therefore US citizens have questioned why their government is not taking the pandemic more seriously when it has a higher death rate than both their invasion of Vietnam and the 9/11 terrorist attack in New York.

The response to COVID-19 draws stark contrast between socialism and capitalism, but to leave it as this is incredibly oversimplistic. New Zealand has been one of, if not the most, successful capitalist countries in dealing with the virus partially for geographic reasons but also because the New Zealand Government was willing to fully lockdown the country and more importantly, fund workers' wages and other business expenses to make sure the lockdown could function well. Countries such as the United States and England have an "austerity capitalism" political doctrine where private enterprise and profit are held as the sole important political consideration. Prioritising the profits of the big corporations put their response, or lack of response, against the interests of the broad masses of people and allowed COVID-19 to run rampant.

Some people said that this epidemic is the most prominent systemic risk test in the public health field that the world has faced since World War II, highlighting the pros and cons of the governance capabilities of capitalism and socialism.

The basic Marxist theory of the state recognizes the state as the instrument of class rule, therefore the state serves the dominant class or classes by furthering their interests. The dictatorship of the bourgeoisie in the capitalist system is exploitative and focused first and foremost on the reproduction of capitalism. This means that the broad masses of working people, the majority in each country, do not have a state that serves their interests, in fact in the ultimate sense, it works against them.

Social welfare and public healthcare programmes under capitalist society benefit the working class (and it is often Communists that won them) but these are implemented only as concessions to ensure the continuation of capitalism. Lenin referred to these reforms as "by-products of the revolutionary movement." This is why no capitalist country has been able to take the necessary measures for a Coronavirus response, such as sweeping nationalisation and capital tax to fund response measures.

Different political paradigms have seen capitalist countries take different measures ranging from a complete disregard of human life to a relatively adequate welfare programme, but they all maintain the exploitation of working people and the continuation of capitalist enterprise. The biggest advantage the developed capitalist countries have had in their COVID-19 responses is simply the funds available for the response effort compared to developing nations (including the socialist countries).

The socialist system has working people at the helm of the state and therefore works in the broad interests of the people, which obviously includes the right to health. Earlier I have discussed some of the institutional specificities of the socialist system that allow this such as the people's army and the neighbourhood committees. Another feature of the socialist system that deserves credit in the COVID-19 response is the people-centred nature of the personnel policy of the Communist Party of China and the Chinese government, including local and provincial officials. This has meant that COVID-19 functioned as a trial by fire where cadre and officials were promoted, reassigned, or removed based upon performance. This meant that the implementation of the COVID-19 response in China was quickly optimised by ensuring there was no dead weight. I think this will have significant and lasting benefits to the system of socialist rule of law with Chinese characteristics.

II. How will the outbreak of this epidemic affect the world configuration?

We are already experiencing significant changes to the world configuration. China and President Xi Jinping have rightly called for increased international cooperation. This is likely to be the case, but at the same time, international cooperation will be equally harmed. We can see this already on a crude level with the majority of countries backing international cooperation, the World Health Organisation, and a public-health based response to COVID-19. Despite a wide variety in social and political systems, these countries also are opposed to the rising Cold War mentality. Serbia, Russia, Pakistan, Venezuela, Zimbabwe, and Cuba are prominent countries who take this position.

On the other end are the countries that serve as the biggest threat to world peace and international cooperation like the United States, Australia and Ukraine. These countries undermine the United Nations and other multilateral institutions, are hostile to China, and militarise the Asia-Pacific to try force it under their influence. New Zealand, the European Union and most other developed countries fall somewhere in the middle, which reflects their competing interests of fealty to US monopoly capital and of their independent economic relations with the rest of the world.

III. The Non-Aligned Movement augmented the influence of the Socialist camp

The competition between the United States and the Soviet Union saw the rise of a strong Non-Aligned Movement of politically diverse countries standing up for peace and multilateralism.

The former Vice-President of Yugoslavia Edvard Kardelj described non-alignment as rejection of a world split into blocs. The 21th century non-alignment, however, is seemingly taking the form of a non-aligned *bloc*. A loose bloc, but a bloc regardless, centred around not only the Non-Aligned Movement, but international bodies such as the Shanghai Cooperation Organisation, Bolivarian Alliance for the People of Our America (ALBA), the African Union and very importantly, the Belt and Road Initiative. These are not organisations to enforce imperialist hegemony like NATO or the Marshall Plan, but neither are they institutions of socialist internationalism like the former Warsaw Treaty or Council of Mutual Economic Assistance (CMEA). These multilateral initiatives rather give the necessary structure to build common development and cooperation free from great power hegemony and imperial *dicta* – the true meaning of non-aligned cooperation.

How the United States will respond to the decline of its hegemony and the rejection of its "world police" policy is a worrying threat to world peace, particularly as the economy continues to decline. The United States and NATO already pursue an aggressive policy against Russia, China, Venezuela and other non-aligned countries politically, diplomatically and economically – Venezuela is at very real risk of a military invasion seeking to return it to the US control. US foreign policy will likely get more desperate and erratic as its dominant position in the world is further replaced by cooperation and non-alignment.

After the outbreak of the COVID-19, Chinese President Xi Jinping made an important instruction, to rely on the masses resolutely in gaining a decisive victory against the epidemic. And China also worked closely with the World Health Organization to promptly and quickly inform the world of the progress of anti-epidemic. However, some politicians, such as those from United States, and the media stigmatized China's efforts repetitively. Some senior US officials publicly accused China of "concealing" the epidemic, and US lawyers even "sued" China for 10 billion yuan, blaming China for failing to contain the COVID-19 and spreading it to the world, making it a costly global pandemic. Other countries have such cases of attempting to pin the blame on China. What is the reason behind this?

In historical and dialectical materialism we can differentiate between necessity and accident. As the People's Republic of China developed it was inevitable that the monopoly-capitalists would increasingly not accept the rise of China, not just as an economic competitor but as a socialist country. COVID-19 has been the "accident" that provided immediate causality for further confrontation with China. No new policy directions towards China have been created in the capitalist countries during the pandemic, old ones have simply been developed. This has the secondary purpose of trying to distract citizens of Western countries from the ineptitude of their own governments in dealing with COVID-19 by blaming it on China, playing off anti-Communist and racist sentiment present in the West.

IV. Suggestions for China and the world to fight against the COVID-19

The primary barrier to a better global response to COVID-19 based on public health principles and cooperation is the continued existence of capitalism in the West. It has poisoned the response to COVID-19 not just because it neglects the health and needs of working people in the capitalist countries, but also because the sanctions and war-mongering of the US imperialists have meant that other nations have found it a lot harder to fight against COVID-19 within their own countries. For example, the Cuban public health ministry was told it could no longer import ventilators from Switzerland because the supplier was bought by a US conglomerate and thus it was illegal under the US blockade. Similar sanctions have affected the COVID-19 fight in countries such as Iran and the Democratic People's Republic of Korea.

Of course, people have wished for the Western capitalist countries to choose the socialist road for over a century and the Western communist movement has travelled a tumultuous path. The key task for the global response is to strengthen the anti-imperialist and peace movement, which in the present scenario means not only standing against sanctions and interventionism as always, but also protecting the multilateral institutions such as the World Health Organisation and the win-win cooperation they enable.

The immense value of the World Health Organisation can be seen by the total hostility shown to it by the United States and the gratitude shown to it by countries such as China, Venezuela, and Iran. It may not be as "trendy" for internationalists to support these measures compared to standing against US interventionism or French nuclear testing, but a peaceful world is no use if most of the population is either dying or dead regardless! This multilateralism, particularly in the areas of public health, is an important part of the peaceful coexistence between capitalism and socialism.

International organisations such as the World Federation of Trade Unions, World Federation of Democratic Youth, and the World Peace Council alongside international cooperation of communist and workers parties have an important role to play in defending peoples' rights and the continued existence of peaceful coexistence itself. Despite the best efforts of the USSR and European People's Democracies for peaceful coexistence and peaceful competition between capitalism and socialism, monopoly-capitalism never ceased its revanchism, culminating in the tragic success of their "peaceful evolution" strategy. We are currently seeing an increased activity of anti-China forces in the US and Europe who seek a similar fate for the PRC. Unity in struggle of world anti-imperialist & peace forces is the keystone in the struggle against interventionism and for the human community of a shared future.

Global Challenge Solved Locally: COVID-19

[Poland] Patrycja Pendrakowska

Edited by Wang Zhen[1]

About the Author

Patrycja Pendrakowska is an analyst on innovations and politics of China. She is the founder of Michał Boym Institute of Asian and Global Studies, and a doctoral candidate at the Faculty of Philosophy and Sociology in the University of Warsaw.

Patrycja Pendrakowska graduated from the sinology (BA), philosophy (BA), sociology (BA), ethnology (MA) and financial law (MA) programs at the University of Warsaw, as well as studied sociology at the Ludwig Maximilian University of Munich. In 2011, she studied migration issues in Nepal, at the Institute for Integrated Development Studies, Kathmandu. She worked at the Security Studies Center, War Studies University from 2016 to 2017. She was the president of Polish-Asia Research Center from 2017 to 2019.

---

1   Zhang Zhen, assistant research fellow of the Academy of Marxism, Chinese Academy of Social Sciences.

Abstract

COVID-19 has proved to have a tremendous impact on the world's politics, economy and society. However, the US government tends to politicize the virus for the domestic purpose, which divide international community in the fight against the COVID-19 pandemic. Although the WHO and Doctors Without Borders make their efforts in this crisis, the COVID-19 became more of a local problem than a global challenge due to lacking of solidarity and cooperation. It is likely that the developing countries will bear most of the economic losses along side the pandemic. Different countries from different political systems background are implementing strict measures to limit the spread of the coronavirus, which shows more effective than those countries that act in a flexible way. Regards to the formulation of anti-epidemic rules, the governments and the public need to build a efficient communication mechanism. In order to minimize the economic and social consequences of any other future epidemics or natural disasters, the policymakers might need to rethink the design of regions, relieving population, developing contactless office and sustainable environment.

I. Introduction

COVID-19 has proved to have a tremendous impact on the world's politics, economy and society. It is still too early to evaluate the long-term consequences of COVID-19 on the way our societies will function, however many ideas on how the post-COVID world will look have already been presented and discussed. One thing is certain though, since January 2020 the virus managed to destabilize the health systems across the globe. Moreover, in the past disease outbreaks proved to be able to change politics, alter societies as well as contributed to different forms of discrimination (Snowden, 2019). Containing the spread of COVID-19 proved to be extremely difficult due to its symptomatic and asymptomatic transmission, and its capability to spread at a high pace. Moreover, the majority of those who contracted the virus experienced only mild symptoms. Still, the medical staff around the world conducts research to develop an appropriate treatment and vaccination. Currently, there are more than 7,273,958 cases of coronavirus in 213 countries, territories, or areas, and 413,372 people have lost their lives (as of June 2020, data source: Doctors Without Borders).[1] As for now there are more cases in the United States (2,064,092) than in any other country.

The origins of the various are a puzzle not only for scientist, but also for politicians, who tend to politicize the virus in order to obtain short term goals on the level of both domestic and international politics. The outcome of the politicization of the disease was the so-called *blame game*. Amid the coronavirus crisis also international organizations setting worldwide standards and procedures have been criticized for their incompetence and partisanship, including the World Health Organization. In fact, pandemic should be a global challenge, but due to the lack of united leadership in the wake of Washington-Beijing rivalry, and a divided international community in the fight against the coronavirus,[2] the disease is mostly handled locally. Moreover, according to some experts like Kori Schake the Deputy Director General of the International Institute for Strategic Studies, the world configuration will inevitably change as the US might lose its status as an international leader. Another important phenomenon involved in the pandemic is its continuous and persistent politicization, which quite often serves domestic purposes, i.e. campaigns and elections. It is also a consequence of difficult economic situations that are linked to social unrests around the world.

The following article aims to investigate the possible consequences of the outbreak of the virus through diagnosing leading problems and challenges for societies. First, it presents the consternations surrounding the role of international

---

1 Doctors Without Borders, 2020, "Facts and figures about the coronavirus disease outbreak: COVID-19," access 12/6/2020 at https://www.doctorswithoutborders.org/covid19.
2 Reuters, 2020, "U.N. chief laments lack of global leadership in coronavirus fight," access 10/6/2020 at https://www.reuters.com/article/us-health-coronavirus-guterres/u-n-chief-laments-lack-of-global-leadership-in-coronavirus-fight-idUSKBN22C3IS.

institutions and organizations amid the COVID-19 pandemic. Secondly, it tackles the debate over the global and local dimension of the disease outbreak as some analysts predict a further decoupling as well as the rising importance of maintaining production within the country. Global pandemic became a threat to many countries of the so-called Global South where production plants are situated. Thirdly, the challenge of social and racial inequalities will be tackled. The virus clearly demonstrated not only social exclusions of the poor, but also racial divisions and stereotypes splitting societies in developed countries. This article also contains subchapters on the way states with different political systems, including liberal and illiberal, are fighting with COVID-19. And a closing part on the potential changes that the pandemic might bring to the working culture and design of public spaces.

II. International Institutions and Organizations

The debate whether international organizations and institutions reacted adequately to the threat of epidemic unfolds as analysts and academicians from various backgrounds share different opinions. On top of that the leading international organization—the World Health Organization became an object of a heated political debate amid tensions between China and USA. President Donald Trump has threatened to pull out of WHO over failed response to the pandemic and accused the director general, Tedros Adhanom Ghebreyesus of not being independent from China.[1] The reaction of president Trump should be perceived in a wider context of the *blame game,* which was unfolding since February/March 2020. The case of WHO's reaction to the first signs of epidemic also became a bone of contention fueled by the rising antagonism between Washington and Beijing. However, opinions on the reaction of WHO on pandemic are quite varied.

---

1 The Guardian, 2020, "Global report: Trump threatens to pull out of WHO over 'failed response' to pandemic," access 4/6/2020 at https://www.theguardian.com/world/2020/may/19/global-report-trump-threatens-to-pull-out-of-who-over-failed-response-to-pandemic.

For example, Alexander White, an assistant professor of sociology and history of medicine at Johns Hopkins University highlights that the response of the World Health Organization (WHO) to COVID-19 was quick: "The response by the WHO to COVID-19 was organized quite quickly. Since 2005, WHO regulations have established protocols and criteria for national health system readiness and also for what constitutes a 'public health emergency of international concern,' or PHEIC. WHO declared a PHEIC for COVID-19 at the end of January, which highlighted the severity of the threat."[1] Others claim that the WHO reacted too slowly on the rumours about the appearance of a new virus in China. According to this scenario (backed up by Trump's administration) the WHO failed to inform on time and thus failed to contain the global spread of the virus, which could be still possible in the very beginning of January 2020. Another important factor eroding the US trust in WHO and China is the alleged lack of adequate information circulation about the disease in the end of 2019. However, due to the fact that the COVID-19 is still a new disease for medical staff and scientists, it is difficult for experts and analysts dealing with political issues on a daily basis to independently evaluate both the alleged level of potential disregard and/or neglect level. What is important is that these uncertainties did fuel further extra politicization.

On the other hand, many organizations are successfully and actively operating transcontinentally in the shade of the WHO. Doctors Without Borders/Médecins Sans Frontières (MSF) is a very good example of a non-politicized organization, which contributes to the fight against the spread of the virus in a reliable and responsible manner. The Geneva-based organization responds to the coronavirus emergency in more than 70 countries and is operating in regions scattered by conflicts and wars. MSF is monitoring the situation in forgotten places around the world, i.e. in Yemen, which since years is being torn apart by war. Since the

---

1   John Hopkins University Hub, 2020, "How Pandemics Shape Society," access 31/5 2020 at https://hub.jhu.edu/2020/04/09/alexandre-white-how-pandemics-shape-society/.

beginning of the epidemic Doctors Without Borders have stressed the difficult situation in refugee camps, conflict scenes around the world and third world countries, where unemployment is on the rise. Moreover, many inhabitants of these places still lack a place they could call home, and under such circumstances social-distancing might be just empty words.

III. Global versus Local

Authorities and organizations around the world claim that the world needs solidarity in fighting the illness rather than rivalry and politicization. The president of MSF highlights that "You will not be safe from COVID-19, until everyone is safe from COVID-19" as the pandemic brings suffering and death to every corner of the world.[1] However, the Global South seems to be much more vulnerable due to the lack of proper healthcare systems, emerging conflicts, economic slowdown and high unemployment rate. Especially touched are refugees, asylum seekers and internally displaced people, who cannot freely social-distance at home.

The epidemic stirred a harsh global political debate, especially after the coronavirus started spreading at a fast pace in the US. Trump's administration blamed China on misinformation, but at the same time it seemed that Washington withheld from taking over a global leadership in the wake of the crisis. As a result, many including Kori Schake the Deputy Director General of the International Institute for Strategic Studies predict that the US will eventually lose its status of an international leader:

The United States will no longer be seen as an international leader because of its government's narrow self-interest and bungling incompetence. The global

---

1 Doctors Without Boarders, 2020, "You will not be safe from COVID-19, until everyone is safe from COVID-19," access 31/5/2020 at https://www.doctorswithoutborders.org/what-we-do/news-stories/story/you-will-not-be-safe-covid-19-until-everyone-safe-covid-19.

effects of this pandemic could have been greatly attenuated by having international organizations provide more and earlier information, which would have given governments time to prepare and direct resources to where they're most needed. This is something the United States could have organized, showing that while it is self-interested, it is not solely self-interested. Washington has failed the leadership test, and the world is worse off for it.[1]

Trump's policy of *America First* seemed to prevail in the White House, being primarily concerned with domestic situations. Simultaneously, China became very active with its *masks* diplomacy becoming one of the most important sources for medical equipment and supplies for the world population. After China managed to control the spread of the virus on its soil Beijing started to promote the Silk Road of Health (健康丝绸之路) as well as added the healthcare aspect to the community of shared future for mankind to its diplomatic portfolio. The rising number of deaths in the USA escalated the rivalry between Washington and Beijing further, as Trump searched for a scapegoat as the situation was slipping out of control. Moreover, the Western countries, including the USA, seemed to be concerned about the growing activity of Beijing. On one hand, China played an important role in delivering medical supplies to European countries in crisis. On the other hand, this activity contributed to a variety of diplomatic spats around the world.

On top of that, many Western policymakers claimed that Chinese model of fighting COVID-19 cannot be implemented in their countries due to differences in political systems and values. Beijing strived to send a unifying message to third countries trying to offer their solutions and medical expertise. In total China has offered medical equipment or medical help to dozens of nations, in Africa, Latin America, East and Southwest Asia as well as Europe. The Council Foreign

---

1 Foreign Policy, 2020, "The Coronavirus Pandemic Will Change the World Forever," access 10/6/2020 at https://foreignpolicy.com/2020/03/20/world-order-after-coroanvirus-pandemic/.

Relations claims that Silk Road of Health might allow China to redeem its national reputation on the international stage. However, different political interests contained the possibility of building a united front towards the epidemic between two world powers the USA and China. European Union decided to find a middle path between these two super-powers.[1]

Generally, the rivalry between world powers was condemned by United Nations Secretary-General Antonio Guterres, who underlined the lack of leadership in the divided international community. He also raised concerns about the inadequate support for poor countries.[2] Despite the strenuous efforts of international organizations COVID-19 became more of a local problem than a global challenge.

Not only Antonie Guterres lamented over the inability to find a common ground on fighting pandemic. Frank Snowden, author of the book Epidemics and Society: From the Black Death to the Present, claims that: "The main part of preparedness to face these events is that we need as human beings to realize that we're all in this together, that what affects one person anywhere affects everyone everywhere, that we are therefore inevitably part of a species, and we need to think in that way rather than about divisions of race and ethnicity, economic status, and all the rest of it."[3]

Some analysts claim that globalization will change its character, becoming more localized and regionalized.

IV. Social Inequalities and social exclusions

The COVID-19 epidemic triggers economic recessions, social unrest and the

---

1   The Council on Foreign Relations, 2020, "Mapping China's Health Silk Road," access 10/6/2020 at https://www.cfr.org/blog/mapping-chinas-health-silk-road.
2   Reuters, 2020, "U.N. chief laments lack of global leadership in coronavirus fight," access 10/6/2020 at https://www.reuters.com/article/us-health-coronavirus-guterres/u-n-chief-laments-lack-of-global-leadership-in-coronavirus-fight-idUSKBN22C3IS.
3   The New Yorker, 2020, "How Pandemics Change History," access 31/5/ 2020 at https://www.newyorker.com/news/q-and-a/how-pandemics-change-history.

feeling of fear all over the world. The pandemic revealed existing social inequalities eroding the economic stability of dozens of countries and international corporations. Millions of people in South Asia lost work as well as their houses or rooms in big cities and had to go back to the countryside. Millions are being challenged by lack of roof, water, food and medical supplies. Currently, when the world's leading broadcasting media concentrate on growing antagonism between the US and China, or focus on economic slowdown, the problems of the Global South are often forgotten. United Nations Deputy Secretary-General Amina Mohammed perceives COVID-19 as a threat multiplier especially for those who are marginalized or live in poor conditions:

We have a health emergency, a humanitarian emergency and now a development emergency. These emergencies are compounding existing inequalities. In advanced economies, we're seeing higher rates of mortality among already marginalized groups. And in developing countries, the crisis will hit vulnerable populations even harder.[1]

One reason for this problem is contracting demand on various products imported i.e. by Western countries from South Asia, Southeast Asia and other places largely dependent on foreign markets. This situation hit factory workers in Bangladesh badly. Many workers cannot afford not to work, but at the same time going back to work in poor conditions can end up in COVID-19 infection. Allegedly a large number of garment factories are not maintaining social distancing and not obeying health safety guidelines .

Amina Mohammed highlighted that the World Bank has estimated that around 49 million people could fall back into extreme poverty. And gender inequalities

---

1   United Nations, 2020, "COVID-19 pandemic exposes global 'frailties and inequalities': UN deputy Chief," access 13/6/ 2020 at https://news.un.org/en/story/2020/05/1063022.

also play an important role as women make up approcimately 60% of the informal economy. At the same time they are earning less and are at a greater risk of falling into poverty. All over the world, similarly in developed and developing countries, women are facing domestic violence. Children are also the ones touched by the pandemic as in many regions of the world they cannot attend schools. Online education is a privilege of the rich, who can afford access to electricity, computers, and a school that provides online lessons. The exclusion of children stemming from poor backgrounds is also an important issue in some countries of the European Union. Another challenge which contributes to rising inequalities is closing down local businesses due to lack of tourists. Already millions of people lost their jobs in this flourishing sector in South Europe or South East Asia. The uncertainty and contracting demand have contributed to the rise of unemployment.

Unfortunately, COVID-19 has also contributed to the rise of racist or discriminatory behaviours towards *strangers*. At first Chinese people were discriminated against as the ones "potentially having the virus." In the US recent protests scattered across the US revealed strong social divisions and the everlasting problem of racism.

V. Political systems facing the epidemic

The COVID-19 epidemic impacts all political systems of the world. It challenges ruling camps in both liberal and illiberal political systems facing policymakers with mighty dilemmas. The actions and methods taken by individual countries, federal states and cities differ a lot. Public health interests were challenged by economic situations. Indeed, taking decisions on lockdowns and later on easing their easing had to be compromised by economic and national interests.

Some liberal democracies like Sweden decided to act in a flexible way. It's policy makers decided to leave a wide scope of freedom to its own citizens and didn't implement a lockdown. However this approach resulted in a number of deaths within the elder part of the society. On the other hand, countries like China (since January 2020) act quickly by testing population and incessantly developing digital surveillance systems to track down potential infections. In these scenarios, quite often control and subordination help to contain COVID-19 in an effective manner. However, some countries i.e. Sweden did avoid taking such measures, which resulted in a higher percentage of infections per 100,000 inhabitants.

Moreover, some democratic states, i.e. South Korea or Israel decided to implement measures that did substantially limit civil liberties or forcefully tracked down infected individuals. This phenomenon using Erich Fromm's vocabulary could be described as an *escape of freedom* (1941), as individuals and societies submitted their scope of freedoms to the authority of the ruling camp. Pursuing Fromm's concept one could also state that European societies melted into *conformity*, which can be described as avoiding genuine *free thinking*. As Fromm claims *free thinking* usually provokes anxiety. In difficult times it might be easier to subordinate, rather than freely discuss and undermine decisions of policymakers that haven't really been debated in the public. Mostly, due to the fear over COVID-19, this transition has been very rash and not consulted between governments and individuals. As Jarosław Kuisz and Karolina Wigura acknowledged silence in the public sphere in the wake of threat doesn't need to mean anything good:

In classical political philosophy it was associated with the danger of despotism (...) Contrary to democracy, characterized by a robust and lively public sphere, in despotism people's interests and activities shift to the private sphere, where they focus on material goods and forget about the community. This threatens democracy, because while people are preoccupied, irreversible changes can be made to the political system.[1]

---

1 The Guardian, "Coronavirus is now contaminating Europe's democracy," access 13/6/ 2020 at https://www.theguardian.com/world/commentisfree/2020/apr/01/coronavirus-contaminating-europe-democracy-viktor-orban-seize-more-power.

Traces of *autocratization* could be also observed in some Central Eastern European Countries as states of emergency and special legal acts were enforced to grant a wider scope of powers to the ruling parties without holding a proper debate (i.e. Hungary). In Poland the lack of procedures and a strategy in the case of pandemic led to a legislative chaos:

Quite often, the speeches of the Prime Minister (executive power) became a source of interpretation of the newly introduced rules. The legal chaos surrounding the epidemic might leave a variety of long-term effects on the Polish civil society. On the one hand it can lead to larger consent to ad hoc fixed decisions and legislations, which in the long run, can lead to recourse from freedom. On the other hand, it can lead to wider criticism of the ruling party, which executes arbitrary power without the social consensus. Indeed, emergencies foster grips of power around the world.[1]

The worldwide trend of emergencies fostering grips of power has been observed and described also by United Nations Deputy Secretary-General Amina Mohammed, who claims that pandemic has contributed to "the erosion of democratic norms that are core to protecting rights and ensuring social cohesion."[2] Indeed, the participation in democratic procedures such as gatherings and demonstrations was limited due to the threat of pandemic. And it doesn't seem that social media offers an adequate solution to that problem in the longer run. They are not specifically policy-oriented, or democracy-oriented as they are listed on the stock exchanges. Their core sense of existence in the capitalist rational – increasing profits from advertising and trading personal data.

---

1 Pendrakowska, P., 2020, "Managing fear and easing lockdown in Poland," *The Observer Research Foundation*, access 13/6/ 2020 at https://www.orfonline.org/expert-speak/managing-fear-and-easing-lockdown-in-poland-67372/.
2 United Nations, 2020, "COVID-19 pandemic exposes global 'frailties and inequalities': UN deputy Chief," access 13/6/ 2020 at https://news.un.org/en/story/2020/05/1063022.

In Europe the COVID-19 pandemic has also contributed to a range of other phenomenons, such as revival of populist Euroscepticism, birth of new conspiracy theories and a stronger commitment to national economy rather than belief in globalization. It became increasingly clear that the world we live in needs proper circulation of verified information and proper citizen education, so that people can effectively distinguish fake news or false allegations.

VI. Space, design, ecology

At the present time when most discussions on COVID-19 are strongly politicized it becomes rather confusing and difficult to imagine a strong united global force, which could help to fight the virus. Certainly, international humanitarian organizations and institutions play a vital role, however their activities funded i.e. by governments have become a subject-matter of international proceedings. What the world might need is an attempt to jointly gather data on best long term solutions, which could minimize the economic consequences of any other future epidemics or natural disasters.

Some experts predict that the COVID-19 epidemic will become a major force enhancing the transformation of urban spaces. Policymakers might need to rethink the design of regions with high density of population. Especially in the slums settlements governors should pay special attention to heat stifles, ventilation and a proper amount of light. Some capital cities still lack of sanitation or piped water supply (i.e. Kathmandu), density of buildings in some districts of Dhaka might prevent fire trucks from reaching gire.

A new climate-friendly approach to mobility is also of value. For example, Brussels aims at lowering transport emissions and plans to give over more spaces to bicycles. For some regions deurbanization might become an answer as it might contribute to creating equal opportunities outside of big capital cities. The threat of COVID-19 already encouraged many professionals to choose home office rather than commute to business centers. This could also contribute to lowering the air pollution in densely populated areas.

Corporations and employers should consider implementation of mechanisms, which could provide better working conditions. Some experts came up with the idea of contactless office, which would enable touchless navigation throughout the working place: "employees could eliminate the need to press communal buttons by using their smartphone to send a command to the elevator or staff coffee machine (in fact, Perkins and Will have such a coffee machine in their new office). Conference rooms could be fitted out with voice-activated technologies to control lighting, audio and visual equipment. Passing through doors or flushing the toilet would require a simple wave, while self-service in office kitchens could become a relic of the past, to be replaced with automation or a dedicated server." Some of these solutions can also be implemented in residential compounds.

Experiences with overcoming challenges related to urban design and working space in the times of pandemic should be shared globally. As we are interconnected and pandemic touches upon developed and developing countries equally it is in the interest of all parties to act jointly. Moreover, a very welcome side-effect of implementing changes to public places design would be strengthening activism and engagement around challenges i.e. climate change and public health. The COVID-19 proved how vulnerable our societies are and might raise awareness about a variety of dangers that are still going to happen in the future. In the longer run COVID-19 might enhance and reinforce grassroot movements and social activism on the local level. What the world needs is more expert knowledge and sustainable governance rather than politicization.

VII. Conclusions

In conclusion, although the COVID-19 pandemic became a global challenge it was mainly solved in a local manner. The lack of leadership from the side of the

USA was certainly one of the main reasons of fighting the COVID-19 on a domestic level—a move which by many commentators is perceived negatively. Rumors arise that the US influences around the world will further erode, as the super-power turns its back to third parties, countries and societies praising *America first* policy. Moreover, in April and May 2020 it became clear that the USA has been hit the worst by COVID-19, and that the government failed to contain the spread of the virus in a reasonable manner. Currently, Washington is facing a major domestic crisis related to the murder of George Floyd and racism. Local treatment of the virus was also sealed by the EU member countries' decision to close down their borders. An unprecedented situation which has never happened before in the history of Schengen countries. COVID-19 revealed particularisms, scepticism and anger across the globe. With this knowledge we should decide how we can prepare for the potential second wave in autumn and to draw long term conclusions, which could become policy recommendations for future generations.

References

Doctors Without Borders, 2020, "Facts and figures about the coronavirus disease outbreak: COVID-19," access 12/6/2020 at https://www.doctorswithoutborders.org/covid19.

Doctors Without Boarders, 2020, "You will not be safe from COVID-19, until everyone is safe from COVID-19," access 31/5/2020 at https://www.doctorswithoutborders.org/what-we-do/news-stories/story/you-will-not-be-safe-covid-19-until-everyone-safe-covid-19.

Foreign Policy, 2020, "The Coronavirus Pandemic Will Change the World Forever," access 10/6/2020 at https://foreignpolicy.com/2020/03/20/world-order-after-coroanvirus-pandemic/.

Fromm, E., 1941, *Escape from Freedom*, New York: Farrar & Rinehart.

John Hopkins University Hub, 2020, "How Pandemics Shape Society," access

31/5 2020 at https://hub.jhu.edu/2020/04/09/alexandre-white-how-pandemics-shape-society/.

Pendrakowska, P., 2020, "Managing fear and easing lockdown in Poland," *The Observer Research Foundation*, access 13/6/ 2020 at https://www.orfonline.org/expert-speak/managing-fear-and-easing-lockdown-in-poland-67372/.

Reuters, 2020, "U.N. chief laments lack of global leadership in coronavirus fight," access 10/6/2020 at https://www.reuters.com/article/us-health-coronavirus-guterres/u-n-chief-laments-lack-of-global-leadership-in-coronavirus-fight-idUSKBN22C3IS.

Snowden, F., 2019, *Epidemics and Society: From the Black Death to the Present* (Open Yale Courses), Yale University Press.

The Council on Foreign Relations, 2020, "Mapping China's Health Silk Road," access 10/6/2020 at https://www.cfr.org/blog/mapping-chinas-health-silk-road.

The Guardian, 2020, "Global report: Trump threatens to pull out of WHO over 'failed response' to pandemic," access 4/6/2020 at https://www.theguardian.com/world/2020/may/19/global-report-trump-threatens-to-pull-out-of-who-over-failed-response-to-pandemic.

The New Yorker, 2020, "How Pandemics Change History," access 31/5/ 2020 at https://www.newyorker.com/news/q-and-a/how-pandemics-change-history.

United Nations, 2020, "COVID-19 pandemic exposes global 'frailties and inequalities': UN deputy Chief," access 13/6/ 2020 at https://news.un.org/en/story/2020/05/1063022.

Compiled Articles

Pandemic of Capitalism and the Treatment Plan*

[Russia] Dmitry Novikov

Compiled by Kang Yanru[1]   *Translated by Li Yi   Finalized by He Jun*

About the Author

Dmitry Novikov (Дмитрий Новиков) was born in Khabarovsk in the Soviet Union (today's Russia) on September 12, 1969. He became a member of the Communist Party of the Russian Federation in 1992, and was elected member and secretary of its Central Committee in 2004. At the 15th Congress of the Communist Party of the Russian Federation in 2013, he was elected deputy chairman of its Central Committee. In 2011 and 2016, Novikov was respectively elected deputy of the State Duma of Russia of the 6th and the 7th convocations, and member of the Parliamentary Group of the Communist Party of the Russian Federation. At the 17th Congress of the Communist Party of the Russian Federation held in 2017, he was elected member of the Central Committee of the Communist Party of the Russian Federation, and was elected member of the presidium and deputy chairman of the Central Committee of the Communist Party of the Russian Federation at the first plenary session of the Congress.

---

* The original title of this article is "Пандемия капитализма и рецепт спасения," digested and compiled from the official website of the Communist Party of the Russian Federation, April 20, 2020, see: https://kprf.ru/party-live/cknews/193531.html.

1 Kang Yanru, assistant research fellow of the Academy of Marxism, Chinese Academy of Social Sciences.

Abstract

The coronavirus pandemic has exposed the strong and weak points of two social-economic systems. China has rapidly brought the coronavirus epidemic under control, while most of the capitalist countries are unable to stop this disaster. China's system ensures that it will effectively stem the spread of the virus. Socialism and the leadership of the Communist Party, which are hated by global capitalists, are the prerequisites for victories in this period. China mobilized human and material resources in a very short period of time, and formulated well-conceived plans to stem the spread of the epidemic. Following the implementation of the plans, millions of people act in a clear and orderly manner without throwing themselves into confusion, and numerous unprecedented moves will be written into history forever.

It is beyond doubt that the victory of China in its battle against the coronavirus represents the victory of socialism. The strengths of socialism and the planned economy have been proved once again. It is hard for capitalist countries to check the spread of the virus because of the underlying reason stemming from the dogma of "new liberalism." The spread of the coronavirus pandemic is transforming the world, and the universal crisis of capitalism is intensified. The effectiveness of socialist system and the ineffectiveness of capitalist model are clearly manifested in the struggle against the coronavirus. Only socialist path can help human beings to get rid of the main threat confronting them – the pandemic of capitalism.

The coronavirus pandemic has become a test to the whole world, as it has revealed the strong and weak points of two social-economic systems. China has rapidly brought the coronavirus epidemic under control, while most of the capitalist countries are unable to stop this disaster.

I. Capitalism's anticommunism lies

The anti-communists mainly criticize socialism for its "low efficiency." They believe that the socialist system is inferior to the capitalist system in every main aspect of social-economic life, and that the socialist policies will inevitably lead to poverty, crisis and collapse, citing the disintegration of the Soviet Union as an "impregnable" argument for their conclusion. It is not accidental that poorly concocted tales run rampant. As it was 100 years ago, proactive anticommunism is still one of the main pillars of capitalist ideology. They view social justice and equality as the main threats to their rule, telling the public horror stories based on the fallacies that "sickles and hammers represent death and hunger." In fact, capitalism does not pay attention to people's well-being at all.

Obviously, only socialism can preclude globalists from plundering the world and manipulating human beings with inhuman rules, in which lies the fear and indignation of the capitalist class. The opponents of socialism shamelessly distort facts out of hatred, and ascribe their own bad habits to a more advanced system. Let's read the following statements: "Socialism and communism cause pain, corruption and decline everywhere. The socialists' eagerness for power leads to expansion, interference and oppression...Following the Bolshevik Revolution in 1917, we noticed the aftermath caused by brutal communist ideology: misery, oppression and death. Communism subjects the inalienable rights of humans to imagined public interests, resulting in the damage to religious freedom, private ownership, freedom of speech and guarantee of life." These views are aired by the incumbent American president, Donald Trump, who probably does not suspect that he made these utterances by following the hysteric logic of Adolf Hitler: "Three kinds of inappropriate and absurd theories are propounded by Marxism: first, it denies the importance of individual; second, it denies the value of private ownership; third, it leads to the destruction of human culture and the crumbling of economy at a higher level (because economy is always predicated on private properties)."

As an indispensable characteristic of capitalist ideology, anti-communism became very active and took on an extreme form when capitalism was mired in a crisis. During the crisis of the 1920s and 1930s, it was the big capital that spawned the monster of fascism. Taking advantage of fascism, big capital attempted to stop the victorious march of the left-wing ideology and effectively destroyed the Soviet Union. We have observed a similar trend today. As capitalism is entangled in various kinds of unsolvable problems, it has once again adopted the protectionist policy to extricate itself from the quagmire and to deceive the working people under the pretext of "protecting traditional values." In such a circumstance, communists are again listed as the main enemies and are affixed with labels such as "antinational force" and "enemy of the motherland." At present, this is a policy typically carried out in the US, Brazil, Poland, Ukraine and many other countries where the political systems do their utmost to serve the interests of big reactionary capitalists.

Anticommunists observe no moral standards. They publicly take advantage of the disaster on humans like a buzzard hovering over its target prey. The spread of the coronavirus clearly proves this point. As China happened to be the first country faced with such a dangerous challenge, the capitalist propaganda machine takes advantage of the incident to attack China's state system and social-economic system. What kind of "falsehood" can Western media not invent? They predicted with a gloating look that China would suffer severe losses, its economy would collapse and a regime change would be unavoidable. *Wall Street Journal*, a mainstream American newspaper, carried a sarcastic report entitled "China Is the Real Sick Man of Asia," in which highly derogatory expressions were found that had been used by the Western colonists to describe China plundered by imperialist powers at the turn of the 20th century.

Such a malicious way of information reporting seemed to have been a success: China was the first country hit by COVID-19, with no experience of fighting the virus. In such a circumstance, even the shortest period of time was highly important, as it could enable people to get materials and goods ready to fight against the epidemic. The densely distributed and highly mobile population complicated the situation further – Wuhan is a metropolis with a population of 12 million, and Hubei

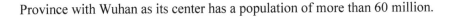

Province with Wuhan as its center has a population of more than 60 million.

II. Effective solution of socialist China

Despite all sorts of slanders, China has successfully withstood the test. With its present system, China ensures that it can effectively stem the spread of the virus. Socialism and the leadership of the Communist Party of China (CPC), which are hated by global capitalists, are the prerequisites for victories in this period. China mobilized the human and material resources in a very short period of time, and formulated well-conceived plans to stem the spread of the epidemic. Following the implementation of the plans, millions of people act in a clear and orderly manner without throwing themselves into confusion.

The following unprecedented moves will be written into history forever: The construction of Huoshenshan Hospital was completed in 10 days to receive patients infected by coronavirus. The hospital occupies an area of 25,000 square meters, and can accommodate 1,000 patients. Three days later, another large-scale hospital – Leishenshan Hospital, was completed. Leishenshan Hospital covers an area of 60,000 square meters, and has 1,600 sickbeds. In a little more than 10 days, China completed the construction of 16 temporary treatment centers boasting the most advanced equipment. An additional 60,000 sickbeds were made available in the city of Wuhan alone. All departments collaborated with each other and worked hard to tackle the challenges. To stem the spread of the epidemic, other provinces across China sent about 43,000 doctors and provided more than 17,000 respirators to Hubei Province. The achievements in China's high technology were fully exploited in the battle against the epidemic. For instance, disinfection robots were widely used in Wuhan.

China regards the battle against the epidemic as a military action. The success of the action is made possible when the Chinese People's Liberation Army takes an active part in it, and when all the Chinese people demonstrate a high level of cohesion and follow strict discipline. People regard the disaster inflicted on the nation as their own misfortune, make concerted efforts in coordination, and have full confidence in the decisions made by the state and its leaders. The action shows high public involvement. Doctors and ordinary people offering themselves as volunteers of the infection centers far exceeded the demand, with CPC members being the most active group of people. At the end of January 2020, Xi Jinping, general secretary of the CPC, appealed to all Party organizations and all Party members, asking them to go to the forefront of the battle against the epidemic. Millions of CPC members answered his call. With their own actions, they refuted the slander of the West saying that the CPC was "a capitalist party" and the CPC members "careerists" caring about their personal gains only.

The coronavirus poses a challenge to more than health. Under the high-pressure environment, all mechanisms in China, including telecommunication, food supply and public security, operate normally as usual, without severe breakdown of any of them. This has been noticed by even foreigners staying in China as well as the Chinese people themselves. For instance, foreigners mentioned the plan of "helping farmers" who had difficulties selling vegetables and fruits because of the health and quarantine measures implemented. In response to this problem, emergency measures were carried out to ensure that the plan of "helping farmers" was launched within just a few days, and the problems were addressed. Likewise, the Russian communists always commit themselves to supporting farmers and agriculture. It was again confirmed at the Oryol International Economic Forum that the support for rural areas is the most important link in safeguarding national security. On April 12, 2020, the Presidium of the Central Committee of the Communist Party of the Russian Federation issued an anti-epidemic statement in which ten anti-crisis measures were proposed. It was stressed in one of these measures that to ensure "the sowing and harvesting of crops," efforts should be made to "urgently adjust the prices of fuels, and fully carry out the plan of supporting the rural areas."

We do not idealize the situation in China. For instance, there exist a small number of officials who neglect their duties, or fail to adapt to the new tempo of work, or cannot make the best decisions rapidly. There are a very few residents who are panic-stricken or people who attempt to seek private gains by taking advantage of the epidemic. The Chinese leaders manage to minimize the negative impacts of these phenomena, and have timely stopped some speculative activities and meted out severe punishment on speculators. With these measures, the shortage of products and health facilities at the onset of the epidemic was relieved, and relevant products were priced in strict accordance with national stipulations. The government strictly controlled the information agenda related to the epidemic, and deleted without delay any false information that could jeopardize public interests. The leaders of the Central Committee of the CPC made it clear that a resolute struggle against discipline violations would be waged. Some high-ranking officials were removed from their offices in the course of the epidemic.

With the implementation of these measures, for the first time since the outbreak of the epidemic in China, there were no newly confirmed cases on March 18, 2020. China displayed the high efficiency of the centralized and unified leadership of the CPC, and the integration of the Party and state organs. As Xi Jinping pointed out: "Our Party was born at a time when China was under the threat of domestic troubles and foreign invasion, grew up through hardships and setbacks, and expanded through tackling difficult problems. Courageously waging struggles and securing victories not only constitute the distinct political character of the members of the CPC, but also demonstrate our political strengths."[1]

III. The victory of China in the battle against the coronavirus is the victory of socialism

The success of China has been recognized by the world. Bruce Alyward, one

---

1   Xi Jinping: "Carry Out All Prevention and Control Work Without Slackening, and Resolutely Secure a Victory in the Battles for Protecting Hubei as Well as Wuhan," *People's Daily*, March 11, 2020.

of the assistant directors-general of the World Health Organization (WHO) and co-leader of the WHO-China Joint Mission on Coronavirus Disease 2019 (COVID-19), said at the end of February 2020 that China's measures for preventing the epidemic from spreading were the only correct measures whose effects have already been proved, and that the Chinese people have demonstrated unprecedented cohesion and unity. His comments were agreed by John Natz, a professor of virology at the Faculty of Medicine at Catholic University of Leuven in Belgium. According to John Natz, the decisive and effective measures adopted by China have won precious time for other countries to take precautionary measures to respond to the spread of the virus.

Even in the US, there are people who appealed to the government to draw on China's experience. James Stavridis, former NATO Supreme Allied Commander Europe, stressed the role played by the Chinese People's Liberation Army in responding to the epidemic in his article to Bloomberg. He thought that the Pentagon should learn how to effectively transfer tasks for civil purpose to the armed forces, and how to coordinate actions between departments to achieve effective collaboration. In response to the article, *New York Times* reluctantly commented that " …outsiders, especially in the West, fixate on China's authoritarian political system, and that makes them discount the possible value and relevance of its decisions to them." However, given the United States' failure in combating the epidemic, the American political elites would not readily acknowledge China's success. The present attitude of Washington is "provocative." The American propaganda tries to deny the way China secured victory in its battle against the coronavirus. Some high-level politicians have called for an investigation into "China's responsibility" in the spread of the virus.

However, nobody can deny the fact that China has responded to the epidemic effectively and controlled the spread of the virus successfully. Some largest political parties in the world, among others, the Communist Party, issued a joint declaration, in which they made a reply in advance to Washington's insinuation. The joint declaration specially pointed out: "We have noticed that China and some other countries have made great progress in preventing and controlling the epidemic. These countries have won time for other countries and are sharing their experience with the international community. We highly appreciate the countries including China, in disclosing timely information about the epidemic, sharing the experience on combating COVID-19 and treating patients in an open, transparent and responsible manner, and providing medical assistance to the best of their capabilities to other countries affected by the epidemic."

There is no doubt that China's victory in its battle against the coronavirus so far is the victory of socialism. Beijing has mastered and adhered to some basic principles of the Soviet Union. The application of these principles enabled the Soviet Union to accelerate industrialization, obtain the victory in the Great Patriotic War, rapidly recover the national economy, make nuclear bombs and send astronauts into the outer space. Under such a model, plan for large-scale national economic development was formulated, strict leadership responsibility system was implemented, and resources were reasonably utilized, with national interests prioritized. The medical and health care system of the Soviet Union, also known as Semashko System, demonstrated the principles of impartiality and equality, under which the public could obtain all kinds of medical assistance free of charge. Based on the principle that the state guaranteed people's health in a centralized and unified way, the medical and health care system attached importance to disease prevention, and always stayed alert to the possibility of the outbreak of epidemic.

IV. Collapse of the delusion of liberalism

The strengths of socialism and the planned economy have been proved once again. With the spread of the coronavirus in other countries, these strengths are becoming increasingly apparent. Although other countries have time to prevent the spread of the virus, the actual situation is indeed depressing, since both the incidence rate and the fatality rate in these countries have exceeded the peak values in China. The Europe and the US are faced with an extremely severe situation. In Italy, a country with a population of just more than 60 million, the number of infected cases exceeded that in China, a country having a population of more than one billion. However, the Western countries have long regarded themselves as examples that other countries should imitate.

The epidemic in capitalist countries is indeed catastrophic, with its underlying reason stemming from the dogma of "new liberalism."

First, the "optimal" integration of the medical and health care system. After the outbreak of the international financial crisis in 2008, the medical and health care systems in Western countries introduced various kinds of mechanisms that would economize on budgets in a most active way. The numbers of hospitals, sickbeds and medical workers all reached what they considered "optimal" levels that "correspond to the average demand." The occurrence of emergency was not taken into account, however. As a result, sickbeds and equipment such as respirators in the hospitals in Italy were in severe short supply. The same situation also occurred in other countries. For instance, the hospitals in Britain refused to accept the patients who cough severely and whose body temperatures are below 37.8 Celsius degrees, because these are considered to be "mild cases." Scientists from Yale University made an astonishing prediction. They warned that one fifth of the American residents, i.e., 60 million people, either have no medical insurance or can enjoy only very low-level medical services. In addition, unable to enjoy paid sick leave or other labor rights, the Americans are worried that they will lose their jobs or face bankruptcy if they receive medical treatment. Their worries were substantiated during the H1N1 influenza epidemic in 2009, when one third of those affected continued to go to work. As a result, the US ranked first among all countries in terms of infected cases and deaths caused by coronavirus.

Next, the inefficient public departments fail to operate properly in times of emergency. The reason, in the final analysis, lies in the values of "new liberalism," in other words, the problems can be attributed to ideas that we should reduce state involvement as much as possible, follow the principle of profit maximization in everything we do, refuse all plans and regulation as they are considered to be "blemishes of totalitarianism." The individualism and the egoism which are based on the social ideology of the capitalist class also play negative roles, which are fully manifested in the crumbling of "European unity." Each country takes actions independently, rather than using the forces of the whole Europe to establish a defensive mechanism. This leads to a self-contradictory and thought-provoking situation: The earliest assistance given to Italy came from China, Cuba and Venezuela, not the European partners.

The COVID-19 pandemic becomes the real "moment of truth," as it reveals what the true value is to human beings, countries and social systems. Being labelled "authoritarian" and "inhuman" by capitalists, socialist countries prioritize people's life and health irrespective of age, gender or race. In "progressive" capitalist society, however, the ugly features of Malthusianism are exposed. Jeremy Warner, a main commentator of *The Daily Telegram*, candidly expressed that "Seen from the purely economic perspective, coronavirus will produce positive influences, because a large proportion of the aged people will be removed from the society." This is just fascism. Patrick Vallance, chief scientific adviser to the British government, proposed the idea of "herd immunity": "As enough of us who are going to get mild illness to become immune to this (virus), it will help us develop herd immunity, so that more people will obtain the immunity to this disease, and reduce further infection." The British government obviously forgets that the aged and the citizens suffering from chronic diseases are the main group of people most vulnerable to coronavirus.

V. Resist the pandemic of capitalism

The profit-seeking free market has always fared poorly in crisis, and the situation is only becoming worse. Although it is hard to predict the scale of the spread of coronavirus, it is obvious that the virus is transforming the world. The universal crisis of capitalism is intensified, and the capitalist class, as usual, will seek a way out through launching a war, bringing disaster to human beings and civilizations, and artificially restoring fascism and anti-human ideology of religious extremism. The only way out for human beings is socialism. The effectiveness of socialist system and the ineffectiveness of capitalist model are clearly manifested in the battle against coronavirus, which is evident to millions of people around the world.

The strike from each crisis further exposes the hazard of the path of liberalism that Russia follows. The fall of oil prices reveals the failure of Russia's diversification policy and Russia's continued reliance on export of raw materials. The coronavirus pandemic demonstrates the great harm of the optimization policy in public sectors. However, the Russian government still refuses to resolutely change the liberal reform initiated by Yeltsin and Gaidar. This means the same decadent ideology is still the basis of the current regime; as a result, there have been absurd accusations against Bolshevik, Lenin and the Soviet state. The lies directed against the Soviet Union usually come from distortion of facts. For instance, some people maintain that the economic growth rate of Russia prior to the October Revolution in 1917 was "astonishing," which ensured that Russia's share of the world's industrial output rise from 5% in 1896 to 5.3% in 1913. In comparison, let's have a look at the achievements of the Soviet government: the Soviet Union's share of the world's industrial output increased from 5% to nearly 20% in just 10 years from 1929 to 1939!

In the ideological construction of the capitalist elites, anti-communism has always been integrated with Russophobia. Through the construction of Yeltsin Center, subsidizing the production of films against the Soviet Union, inciting the hysteria about the Great Famine, and accusing the Soviet Union of launching the Second World War, the capitalist class around the world is scheming to dismember

Russia so that as an independent country it will perish for good. Therefore, defending historical truth is a necessary condition for Russia not to be disintegrated by capitalist plunders.

At present, when global conflicts reach an apex, we must not sit idly for the looming storm without taking any action. In the current circumstance, only China, a country which exhibits solidarity between its people and the government, can continue to march on. However, it is impossible for capitalist world which is built on a decadent basis mixing "new liberalism" with pseudo-patriotism of anticommunism and monarchism to achieve unity. Only socialist path can help human beings to get rid of the main threat confronting them – the pandemic of capitalism.

COVID-19: the Complete Failure of a System*

[France] Bruno Guigue

Compiled by Zhang Jinling[1]   Translated by Li Yi   Finalized by He Jun

> ## About the Author
>
> Bruno Guigue, a French political scholar, was born in Toulouse, France in 1962. He served as a senior civil servant in France, and is a professor of philosophy at University of Reunion Island (Université de La Réunion). He mainly specializes in the studies of international politics.

---

*   On February 7, 2020, *The World* (*Le Monde*) carried an editorial that waged an unfounded attack against China. The editorial claimed that doctor Li Wenliang, who died because of being infected by coronavirus, was a symbol of "the failure of the Chinese system." Since the outbreak of the epidemic, such a kind of view prevailed in the media and political discourse of the entire Western world. On March 9, Professor Guigue posted his criticism of this view on his Facebook account. His criticism was later widely reprinted on the websites of many organizations (some media agencies included) except for mainstream French media agencies, under the annotated title of "COVID-19: The Failure of a System," and produced positive influences among large numbers of netizens. See: Bruno Guigue, "Covid-19: la faillite d'un système," March 29, 2020, https://www.egaliteetreconciliation.fr/spip.php?page=article&id_article=58503#forum. – *Zhang Jinling*

1   Zhang Jinling, research fellow of the Institute of European Studies of Chinese Academy of Social Sciences.

Abstract

In his article, Guigue expresses his positive attitude towards the efforts and effects of China's battle against the epidemic, and delivers a powerful counter-blow to the criticisms of China's system by the Western media. The article makes it clear that the Chinese system has the decision-making, mobilization, implementation and error-correction capabilities to respond to an epidemic, although it does not directly air this view. To him, these are where the strengths of the Chinese system lie.

The author criticizes France and other European countries for losing their roles and functions as "state." The European states today have not only been abducted by financial capitals and lost their fiscal capabilities, but also abandoned their sense of responsibility for the people. The Western countries have lost the awareness of self-reflection and the capability to take actions.

The article argues that the Chinese system is not the totalitarian dictatorship system that the Western countries believe it is. Instead, it is a reliable system, although it is not perfect. The COVID-19 pandemic indeed reflects the failure of a system. However, it is the present system of the Western countries that has failed, rather than the Chinese system.

People may have read, seen or heard the following remarks: "The Chinese regime has collapsed," China "is on the verge of collapse," "The state system is precarious as if it were standing on the edge of an abyss," "finds itself under attack from all quarters," "admits its failure," and "Everything will never be the same."

In fact, one thing is for sure: everything will never be the same. Such a remark is well-founded: China has brought the epidemic under control within just two months. Those ill-intended people would say that this is not true: the number is falsified, and the epidemic will rebound. But international experts will give an opposite answer, as the facts are self-evident. Today, the daily number of newly infected cases in other parts of the world is more than 50 times as large as that in China. More than 70,000 patients out of the

80,000-plus cases recorded in China since January 2020 have been cured. The restrictions on travel are being lifted, and the economic activities are restarted.

We know such a reality saddens a large number of China's enemies active in the media in the world of freedom. They have to adapt to such a reality, however. China has successfully achieved what cannot be done in any other country: it has stemmed the epidemic through large-scale social and national mobilization. China has entered "a state of war" ever since it reported coronavirus to the World Health Organization on December 31, 2019. Starting from January 23, 2020, China unprecedentedly ordered a lockdown involving 50 million people – a measure that slowed the spread of the epidemic.

On February 8, 2020, President Xi Jinping, wearing a face mask, announced on television that "a people's war on epidemic prevention and control" would be launched. Thousands upon thousands of volunteers flocked to Hubei Province, and dozens of hospitals were completed in just a few weeks. Thousands of teams were sent to track infected patients and find out their contact with other people. To cite an example: Towards the end of the Chinese New Year holiday, 860,000 people returning to Beijing were required by the government to isolate themselves at home for two weeks. The city of Beijing mobilized 160,000 people to serve as entrance guards of residential quarters to ensure compliance with the order.

If the pandemic is subsided, it is not because the Chinese people have turned their prayer wheels, but because they have spared no efforts to constrain the virus. In Europe, people criticize China for passing the buck to others, and "prioritizing economic development." Meanwhile, COVID-19 is spreading rapidly across Europe. In 2009, the H1N1 flu virus that appeared in Mexico and the EU countries infected 1.6 million people, and costed the lives of 284,000 people around the world. In the face of this pandemic, Washington is so "extraordinary" that it can do nothing about it, while the Western media are more willing to cast their eyes elsewhere.

Today, it has to be admitted that the socialist system in China again exhibits its superiority while our system does not work, because a state is still needed to cope with such a threat. But where is our state? Does it prioritize public health? Even if it is keen on destroying existing hospitals, is it capable of building new ones?

In a country where public properties are negative, public services are privatized or destroyed, and the "state" voluntarily allows itself to be a hostage to the financial sector, are we capable of achieving 10 percent of what the Chinese have done? It is true that Beijing does not adopt the model of "new liberalism," the banks in China are subject to the government, the public properties account for 50 percent of the wealth of nationals, the country is responsible for the results, 800 million netizens can assess the state's capabilities of handling problems, the country understands that it should be responsible for the national interests, and that it cannot be continued unless it can deliver practical performances instead of paying lip service. Is this system a totalitarian dictatorship?

This is a very strange dictatorship system, under which debates are going on, mistakes are denounced, demonstrations are held from time to time, and systems are open to criticism. Is it a totalitarian system just because it ordered a lockdown for a large population – although all experts admit this is the only effective measure? Probably it is not a perfect system, yet it operates normally and spots its own mistakes. In comparison, in our country, self-satisfaction replaces self-criticism, slandering others substitutes for bearing responsibilities, and long-existing eloquent empty talk takes the place of effective actions.

The editorial writer of *Le Monde*, who is a leading scientist, was right when he said: "This is a complete failure of a system." The system that has failed completely, however, is not the one in the minds of people.

COVID-19: Catalyst for World Crisis and China's New Role*

Research Group on "China and World Power Landscape,"

Latin American Council of Social Science

Compiled by Lou Yu[1]   Translated by Li Yi   Finalized by He Jun

---

About the Author

Latin American Council of Social Science (CLACSO in short in Spanish) is a non-governmental organization accredited by the UNESCO. Established in 1967, it is dedicated to research in the fields of social sciences and humanities. It is one of the three major social science research institutes in Latin America, with the other two being the Latin American Faculty of Social Sciences and the Economic Commission for Latin America and the Caribbean, the United Nations. At present, CLACSO has 680 member institutes, social sciences research institutes and post-graduate bases in 51 countries including the US, Canada, Germany, Spain, France, Portugal, and Latin American countries.

---

*   The original title of this article is "Catalizador de la crisis mundial y el nuevo papel de China," and is originally carried in the column of "Focus on the Pandemic: Social Observation of Coronavirus (Pensar La Pandemia: Observatorio Social del Coronavirus)" by Latin American Council of Social Science, May 4, 2020, see: https://www.clacso.org/covid-19-catalizador-de-la-crisis-mundial-y-el-nuevo-papel-de-china/.

1   Lou Yu, assistant research fellow of the Institute of Latin American Studies of Chinese Academy of Social Sciences.

Abstract

Following the outbreak of the COVID-19 pandemic, a number of changes are taking place, including the formation of a new global geopolitical landscape, the questioning on the globalization of "new liberalism," and the change of technological paradigm. De-globalization, the fourth industrial revolution and the new model of accumulation created by China are becoming a new trend and new characteristics. Since the outbreak of the pandemic, the world power and its new landscape in Latin America demonstrate that China today has set an example for Latin America and even the whole world. Latin America is in urgent need of abandoning the colonial perspective of Europe and the US, and constructing a perspective of "looking at China based on Latin America itself."

The outbreak of COVID-19 triggers a large-scale discussion on its impact on the global power landscape. The global power landscape has undergone constant changes since 2000. In particular, the financial crisis that occurred in 2008 has profoundly changed the global landscape. The world, which has not yet fully recovered from the heavy losses inflicted by that economic crisis, has been plunged into another crisis caused by the COVID-19 pandemic since January 2020. It is no doubt that the pandemic has become a catalyst or accelerator for adjusting world landscape.

I. New global geopolitical landscape

What overall impact will the COVID-19 pandemic make? What influences will different measures that have been taken in response to the pandemic exert on the operation of capitalism and the global power landscape? It is impossible for these influences to fully and accurately manifest themselves at the present stage. The age in which we are living is filled with all kinds of uncertainties. COVID-19 is just like a "changing card." Its appearance at least made us feel certain about one thing: The world has changed, and the world we bade farewell to in December 2019 no longer exists.

Following COVID-19 are a series of changes, such as the formation of a new global geopolitical landscape, the questioning on the globalization of "new liberalism," and the change of technological paradigm. Meanwhile, a new model of accumulation is attracting universal attention worldwide. This model of accumulation is constructed on the basis of fast-changing technological innovation and an entirely new relationship of "citizens – government – market," which is unlike the Western social engineering. The benchmark of this model of accumulation is mainly found in Asia, with China being the most typical one. In view of such a change, it is predictable that the geopolitical competition between old developed countries and emerging powers will be intensified in Latin America and the Caribbean Region.

After a fragile truce on trade war was reached between China and the US (against the backdrop of a technological competition and geoeconomic war), the geopolitical competition between the two countries is intensified amid the pandemic, in particular, in the field of public opinions. For instance, there were statements that China should be "held accountable" for the COVID-19 pandemic sweeping across the world, and that the COVID-19 pandemic is spelling the end of China as a major power ("China's Chernobyl Moment"). In just a few days, however, the Western countries' accusations were powerfully refuted by the realities. China actively conducts international collaboration, playing an important role in the global fight against the pandemic (Of course, Russia and Cuba are also among the countries providing international collaboration).

In stark contrast with China, the US and the EU have delivered disappointing performances. The original intention of establishing the EU is on the verge of collapse. The EU initially failed to take any unified measures in response to the pandemic, and then its delayed apology did nothing to save its image as an organization that is in immediate danger. The cooperation of member states of the EU was absent at a time when the EU was most in need of joint actions and unified coordination.

In the face of the spread of the COVID-19 epidemic in the US, the American government's irresponsible responses have damaged its own image. Preaching nationalism and anti-globalization, the American government acted obstinately, taking more radical actions and frequently accusing several multilateral organizations. Driven by the US, these organizations were established in the wake of the Second World War and are an integral part of the American hegemonic system. The organization recently accused by the US is the World Health Organization (WHO).

The COVID-19 has accelerated the consolidation of China's status in the world stage. As early as 2001, the US regarded China, a giant in Asia, as a strategic competitor, and adopted a series of measures to contain China while developing cooperative relations with it. Later, with the constant development of the BRICS mechanism formed from 2008 to 2009, China has purchased less and less American national debts, and began to buy foreign enterprises around the world. Moreover, in 2013, China initiated the Belt and Road Initiative, which is regarded as a response to the Trans-Pacific Partnership (TPP). All the above measures form part of the war of reconstructing the world system. The relations between China and the imperialist America go from bad to worse in this war which is turning increasingly into a tangled and fragmented warfare, and the geopolitical conflict is intensified correspondingly.

II. De-globalization, the fourth industrial revolution, and the new model of accumulation created by China

It is predicted that nationalism in the most conservative sense will rebound after the end of the COVID-19 pandemic. Of course, there were already signs of this trend prior to the outbreak of the pandemic. The main indicators of the globalization of "new liberalism" began to show a declining tendency several years ago and the crisis from 2008 to 2010 was its turning point. From then on, the international trade and foreign direct investment began to slow down, and they have not yet recovered their vitality.

Through comparing the effectiveness of the measures adopted by different countries in the battle against the COVID-19 epidemic, we find that Asian countries, especially China, play a positive role in leading and effectively implementing a new biotechnological paradigm, with obvious positive effects. China and some other Asian countries compare favorably with the countries in other parts of the world in the fields of government organization capacity, application of cleaning and disinfection technology, and public health. This has also been proved by South Korea and Vietnam. In contrast, the incompetence of most developed Western countries in rising to the challenge posed by the pandemic is also obvious to all.

Having implemented reform of the socialist market economy at a still higher level, China is further promoting economic development at a faster-than-expected speed, demonstrating the effectiveness of its reform of the socialist market economy. China has superior material conditions to guarantee that it can develop economy with almost no obstruction. The China model is a new variant of the planned economy, whose operation is almost free from the bottleneck restrictions caused by finance, external conditions and productive capacity. The advanced ergonomics and social engineering in China are based on such a model, whose superiority has been tested in this battle against the pandemic. In addition, this new variant of the planned economy is the antithesis of the excessive financialization of economy. At present, excessive financialization no doubt has aggravated the moral crisis and intellectual degradation in the West.

It should be stressed that the Western countries adopted tightening policies in the wake of the financial crisis in 2008. At present, however, the tightening policies and the policy of restricting public spending are creating obstacles to the liberal Western governments (except for a few countries including Germany) in effectively responding to the crisis. Unlike Western countries, China did not adopt tightening policies, and it has also achieved positive results in resolving the classic dilemma caused by the market economy and socialism. Of course, China is still confronted by environmental, social and political problems. It has issued a series of policies to address these problems, including making domestic demand the main engine driving economic development, regulating foreign direct investment, and keeping to the path of socialist construction with Chinese characteristics, without restricting itself to following the common models of development.

On the one hand, the conflicts between those advocating the cooperation between the European and American continents and those upholding globalism are increasingly prominent; on the other hand, China proactively "connects" itself with multi-polarization to play a leading role in the world. In the face of the outbreak of a pandemic worldwide, China actively provides international assistance and further promotes infrastructure construction, and the latter is the most distinctive characteristic of the Belt and Road Initiative. These Chinese projects have made progress even in Europe.

The crisis triggered by the COVID-19 pandemic shows that it is necessary to "get rid of" the globalization based on "new liberalism" so as to handle the challenge posed by the global pandemic, or at least make swift responses. For many years, China has been designing its own model of development. Of course, China has no intention of persuading other countries to accept the universality of its development model. No matter what kind of development model a country adopts, it is necessary to contemplate thoroughly the choice and figure out which can be handed over to the market and which cannot. Obviously, health, education and some specific economic sectors cannot be handed over to the "invisible hand," otherwise, dear prices would be paid in terms of the economy, society and labor force even in the middle period. This is a bitter lesson left to us by the COVID-19 pandemic. Over the past decades, most countries in the world have embraced the "new liberalism" model. However, the COVID-19 pandemic has struck a heavy blow to this model.

It is known to all that globalization is stagnating, and the competition of capital is intensifying. The two are connected and influence each other, and are triggering a series of conflicts, dilemmas and challenges. For instance, the peripheral economic structure may possibly suffer losses because of excessive financialization or excessive reliance on the economy of the northern hemisphere. The relationship between labor and capital is increasingly tense. Many countries attempt to resume the industrialized production in some fields, which will inevitably aggravate more conflicts worldwide. The value creation model of the past is out of date (which leads to great damages to the value), and new value creation models have emerged. Meanwhile, thanks to the fourth industrial revolution, the semi-peripheral countries are plunged into the dilemma of "accession" or "being absolutely peripheralized," which may lead to the reappearance of the forces of anti-hegemonism.

III. World power and its new landscape in Latin America

China today has set an example for Latin America, or perhaps even the whole world. Through geopolitical cooperation, China has obtained leadership in the world, and is poised to bear the economic costs required by this leadership at any time. China's new development model based on domestic demands will inevitably impact the economy of Africa and Latin America. As the crisis associated with the Western liberal and democratic model and the development model it imposed on its peripheral area deepens, an entirely new map of conflicts is taking shape.

In the face of the pandemic, Latin America is under double attacks caused by both new and old crises. On the other hand, Latin America should rethink and timely adjust a number of policies, such as those concerning agricultural production, in particular, agricultural exportation, and giving assistance to health and education, improving productive capacity, diversifying industrial structure, and promoting integration process.

For Latin America, crisis comes with opportunity. To make use of the opportunity, Latin America must carefully plan and work out its strategic policy towards China rather than letting things take their own course and eventually becoming an appendage to China. The risk lies in that during the global crisis, the extractive export of raw materials will probably be increased further, while the diversification reform of industrial structure of domestic market in Latin America will probably stagnate.

Latin America is a region composed of many independent countries. It is in urgent need to reiterate this view, and think about the development of Latin America based on this view. There is also the need to always maintain the critical thinking of Latin America. Finally, Latin America is in urgent need of abandoning the colonial perspective of Europe and the US, and constructing a perspective of "looking at China based on Latin America itself."

Contributors

Jiang Hui

Vice president of the Chinese Academy of Social Sciences (CASS), a member of the Leading Party Members' Group of the Chinese Academy of Social Sciences, director of the Institute of Contemporary China Studies (at the level of vice minister), director of the Academy of Marxism, research fellow and tutor for doctoral candidates. He is concurrently the executive director of the Research Center of Xi Jinping Thought on Socialism with Chinese Characteristics for a New Era, director of the Research Center for Theoretical System of Socialism with Chinese Characteristics, and deputy director of World Socialism Research Center. He is deputy director of the Scientific Socialism Institute of China, and deputy director of the Chinese Society of History of Communist Party of China. He is one of the "Young and Middle-aged Experts with Outstanding Contributions," one of the recipients of "Special Government Allowances of the State Council," one of those supported by "One Hundred, One Thousand and Ten Thousands of Talent Program," a leading talent in philosophy and social sciences under the national special support program for high-level talents (ten thousand talents program), one of the theoretical talents and cultural masters of the "Four Batches," and the main expert of the CPC Central Committee's Project for the Study and Development of Marxist Theory.

Jiang Hui has long been engaged in the study of Marxist theories, scientific socialism and international socialist movement, socialism with Chinese characteristics and socialism in contemporary world. He has published many monographs and translated works, served as the chief editor of some works, and published more than 200 papers on important newspapers at the central level and prestigious academic periodicals. He has long been in charge of key research projects sponsored by the National Social Science Fund of China, the CPC Central Committee's Project for the Study and Development of Marxist Theory, and major research projects of the Chinese Academy of Social Sciences, and has obtained positive results. He has important and extensive influences in the research fields of international communism and scientific socialism, world socialism, and innovation and development of Marxism in the 21st century.

Research Center of Xi Jinping Thought on Socialism with Chinese Characteristics for a New Era at Chinese Academy of Social Sciences

Established on December 29, 2017, it is one of the 10 research centers (institutes) on Xi Jinping Thought on Socialism with Chinese Characteristics for a New Era established with the approval of the Central Committee of the Communist Party of China. Its main functions are to specialize in the research of Xi Jinping Thought on Socialism with Chinese Characteristics for a New Era, and organize the publishing of theoretical articles on the three newspapers and one periodical under the CPC Central Committee (i.e. *People's Daily*, *Guangming Daily*, *Economic Daily* and *Seeking Truth*), undertake subject researches and hold academic seminars by bringing into play the distinctive characteristics and advantages of the Chinese Academy of Social Sciences. In recent years, the Center has played an important role in conducting systematic, in-depth and comprehensive study of and giving publicity to Xi Jinping Thought on Socialism with Chinese Characteristics for a New Era.

World Socialism Research Center, Chinese Academy of Social Sciences

In 1994, six ministries and commissions under the Central Committee of the

Communist Party of China organized a research group to track and study socialism in other countries. The Chinese Academy of Social Sciences established a non-entity research organization – World Socialism Research Center, Chinese Academy of Social Sciences in 2001 for the same purpose. Through more than 20 years of development, World Socialism Research Center has extensively united domestic and international forces in this field of study, and produced a series of authoritative, branded and foresighted research findings on a broad range of significant historical and realistic issues including the theoretical trend of thought of world socialism movement, and fostered and guided a large number of domestic and international talents specializing in world socialism.

Research Department of Overseas Marxism, Academy of Marxism, Chinese Academy of Social Sciences

The Research Department mainly studies the emergence, evolution and basic thoughts of Marxism in the contemporary world, world socialism and related theories, trends of thought and schools of thought. Under the Research Department are three research offices that study theories of foreign communism, foreign left-wing ideologies, and Western Marxism respectively. The Research Department has reasonably distributed academic disciplines, powerful overall research strength, extensive international academic exchanges and fruitful research results. In recent years, centering on the priorities of the Chinese Academy of Social Sciences, the Research Department has made outstanding contributions in playing its roles as a think tank and advisory body of the CPC and the State.

This book is the result of a co-publication agreement between Contemporary China Publishing House (China) and Paths International Ltd (UK)

Title: China's Fight Against the COVID-19 Epidemic: Its International Contribution and Significance in the Eyes of the World
Editor-in-Chief: Jiang Hui
Associate editors: Xin Xiangyang, Gong Yun
Edited by Li Ruiqin, Yu Haiqing, etc.
ISBN: 978-1-84464-676-0
Ebook ISBN: 978-1-84464-677-7

Paths International Ltd
www.pathsinternational.com
Published in the United Kingdom

CPSIA information can be obtained
at www.ICGtesting.com
Printed in the USA
LVHW061321180222
R17171700001B/R171717PG710826LVX00002B/1